THE 3-DAY
RESET

Restore Your

Cravings for

Healthy Foods

in Three Easy,

Empowering Days

• • •

POOJA MOTTL

SEAL PRESS

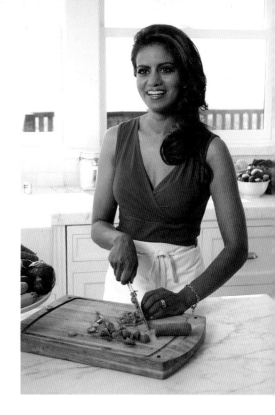

THE 3-DAY RESET
Restore Your Cravings for Healthy Foods
in Three Easy, Empowering Days
Copyright © 2014 Pooja Mottl

Published by
Seal Press
A Member of the Perseus Books Group
1700 Fourth Street
Berkeley, California
sealpress.com
The3DayReset.com

Photography Credits: All photos © Pooja Mottl except: pages ii, v, 12, 80, 202, and 255 © Austin Goldin; page
16 (bottom) © Michelle Kiefer; page 38 © Jonathan Bregel and Khalid Mohtaseb; page 312 © Gregg Delman.

Library of Congress Cataloging-in-Publication Data

Mottl, Pooja, author.
    The 3-day reset : restore your cravings for healthy foods in three easy,
empowering days / Pooja Mottl.
        pages cm
    ISBN 978-1-58005-527-7 (paperback)
1. Natural foods—Health aspects. 2. Lifestyles—Health aspects. 3.
Health behavior—Decision-making. 4. Cooking (Natural foods) I. Title. II.
Title: Three-day reset.
    RM237.55.M68 2014
    641.5'637—dc23

                                2013047081

9 8 7 6 5 4 3 2 1

Cover and interior design by Domini Dragoone
Cover photo © Austin Goldin
Printed in China by RR Donnelley
Distributed by Publishers Group West

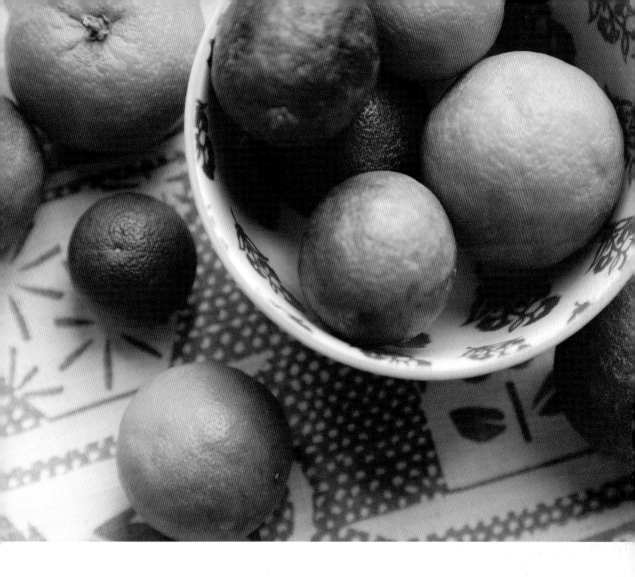

Dedication

For Trevor, Valentina, and Benny:

Gratitude. Peace. Love. Mindfulness.

Contents

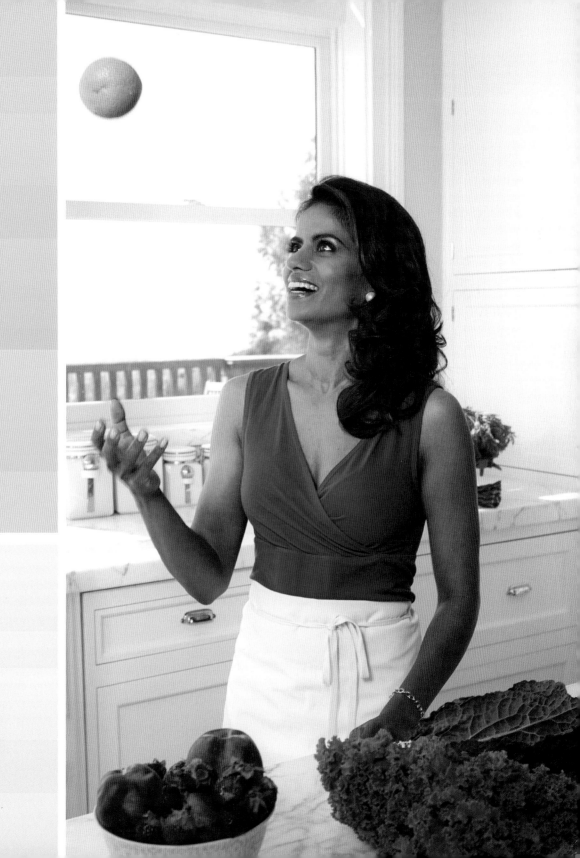

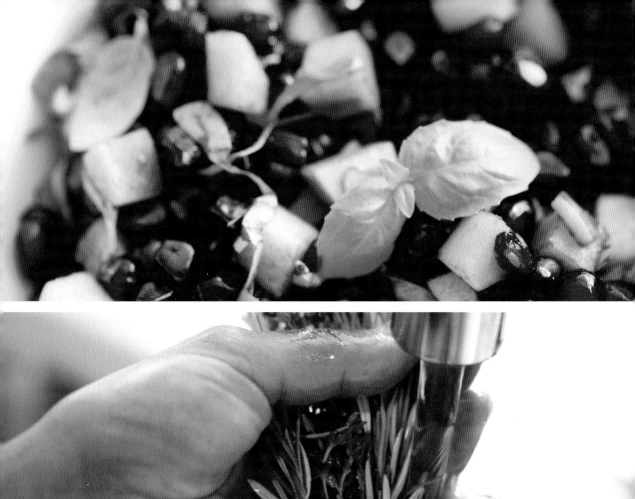
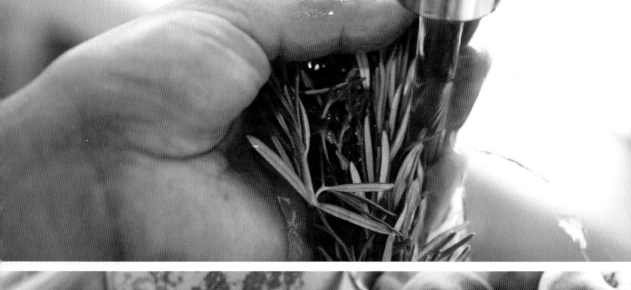
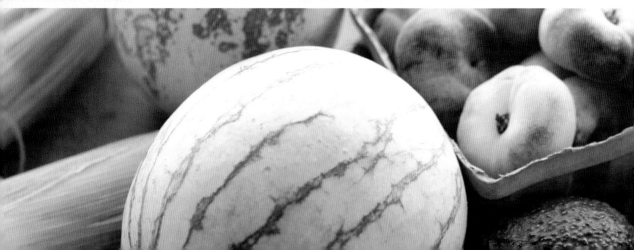

Introduction

"You picked the veggies, rice, and beans over a piece of pizza?
You've got to be crazy! How do you have the willpower and discipline?"

"I got you a cappuccino, but there's sugar in it so I know you won't
drink it. You've got to be the healthiest eater I know! I don't think
I could ever be that disciplined."

Over the years, these are some of the hundreds of remarks and questions I've fielded from clients, friends, and family alike. People want to know my "secrets." They want to know why I crave nourishing foods and why healthy eating comes so easily to me. They want to know how they, too, can figure out what the healthiest foods and drinks really are among the ocean of choices at the supermarket. They want to look good and feel good by eating right.

The truth of the matter is that healthy eating need not be confusing, nor should it require rules, restrictions, or sacrifices in flavor. In fact, we are all biologically hardwired to *crave* healthy foods. All we need to do is restore ourselves back to what comes naturally. In other words, we need a Reset.

The 3-Day Reset (3DR) offers a revolutionary way to do just that.

By focusing on ten of the most common ingredients, foods, and dishes available to us every day, 3DR restores us to our true, natural relationship with healthy food—a relationship that makes eating healthily effortless and delicious. It does this by changing the way we *define* healthy food and how we *experience* its flavor using a self-empowering, bite-sized methodology I call a "Reset." In doing so, it allows us to make eating right a long-term, enjoyable part of our lives.

3DR is the ultimate anti-diet book and is nothing short of a breakthrough. It's the iPhone of healthy eating—clean, clear, easy, and once you use it, you'll find it hard to go back to eating the way you used to.

The magic behind 3DR is in the concept of "Resetting"—all we need to do is reset our connection with food. Just like you reboot your computer to allow it to restore itself, 3DR restores you to a relationship with healthy food that is in concert with your body's chemistry. You'll get back to the basics, get back to eating and loving food the way Mother Nature intended, and forget everything else that's been thrown at you in the past. 3DR overhauls the way you're currently thinking about, buying, and consuming food.

With this book, you can toss out many of the diet books you've acquired over the years because you'll no longer need them. 3-Day Resets gives you *tools*, not rules, and puts you in the driver's seat when it comes to your food choices. You can also stop listening to a lot of the advice doled out by some nutritionists and food experts who have no problem telling you *what* foods to eat, while failing to make them foods you *want* to eat. 3DR celebrates only what's delectable.

3DR works by not only teaching you about healthy food, but also by allowing you to taste, smell, see, and touch it too—a powerful and effective dual approach for making long-term, sustainable change.

The 3-Day Reset is nothing short of life changing and eye-opening. It changed my life, and it can change yours too. If you're someone who wants to eat healthier but haven't yet found a way to eat the foods you know you should, you've come to the right place.

My Journey to The 3-Day Reset

Long before I devised The 3-Day Reset, I didn't know how to navigate the supermarket, nor the kitchen. And I certainly didn't find healthy food delicious—I'd take a greasy hamburger over a tossed salad any day! I thought eating healthily meant I had to eat tofu, lots of bland and uninspiring salads, and less of everything that actually tastes good.

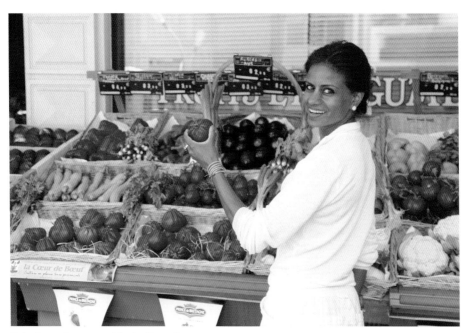

Enjoying a farmstand in Antibes, France

And then it all changed.

My story begins in Ann Arbor, Michigan, where I was born and raised. Growing up, I never thought about the food I was eating. I just ate what my parents brought into the house. I was lucky in that they cooked a lot and didn't buy much soda pop or candy, but there was plenty of processed food: Eggo waffles, Pepperidge Farm Sausalito cookies, Campbell's Chunky soup, and Pop-Tarts were constant staples in our kitchen. I was never terribly overweight, but I was pudgy sometimes, and I had a weakness for Burger King Whoppers, A&W Root Beer Floats, and McDonald's Shamrock Shakes.

For a long time, this worked out okay. In middle school I began playing team sports, which helped my body deal with all that bad food I was eating. By the end of high school, I was a three-sport varsity athlete—golf, tennis, and volleyball—and I felt fit, strong, and healthy. I ate what I wanted when I wanted to and didn't give it a second thought.

But that didn't last. As I grew older, I found I couldn't sustain that vitality of my teenage years, but I didn't know why. It wouldn't be until college and several years after graduation that I would finally start making the connection between food and the way

> Just like you reboot your computer to allow it to restore itself, each 3-Day Reset restores you to your most fundamental, human, natural relationship with food. You'll get back to the basics, back to eating and loving food the way Mother Nature intended.

I looked and felt. After burning the midnight oil enough as an economics major at the University of Michigan to earn me the grades I needed to get a coveted Wall Street investment banking job upon graduation, I found myself overweight, stressed, and exhausted. I still remember a night when I was stuck in the office well after the sun went down and spent hours chowing down on junk foods in an unsuccessful bid to get a boost of energy and focus. I left that night, my office trash bin full of wrappers, feeling bloated, disgusting, and burned-out, my project still unfinished. What I was choosing to eat and my lifestyle in general had to change. The food I was eating was hurting me, not helping me.

I had always been the type of person who wanted to have boundless energy to tackle the world, and I wanted to do whatever it took to look and feel my best. I wanted to feel the same way I had when I was younger—athletic, fit, and happy. But in the real world, it was becoming a challenge. I tried to find good examples in my female friends and coworkers but realized they too were struggling. In an effort to lose weight, most of my friends were skipping meals or eating very little. My office mate would show up in the morning with an extra-tall latte and a brownie, which she'd sip and munch on for most of the day in an effort to ward off the need to "eat a meal." Another ate only soup for lunch, another handfuls of jellybeans and not much else. Since I had no idea what eating healthily meant, or how to cook for myself, I fell into a similar trap. For at least a year I remember surviving on just smoked salmon and fruit chews.

I also tried the standard diets. Since nutritional advice was splattered all over the pages of women's and fashion magazines, I thought it high time I gave the "1/2 cup of cottage cheese" and "3 oz chicken breast" type of diets a whirl. I figured if there was so much advice out there, these people probably knew what they were talking about. I tried journaling about my food. I tried low-carb, low-fat, low-calorie deprivation diets and detox plans, but they all seemed so brutal, so hard, and not the least bit tasty. Most importantly, *I couldn't stick with them.* Nothing was sustainable. I didn't feel that much healthier or energetic, and worst of all, eating this way didn't feel at all natural. Besides, I was busy! I didn't have the time to dedicate to food and my health—I was too busy trying to further my career, maintain a social life, and keep up with the daily demands of a very busy adulthood.

Luckily, an epiphany was just around the corner. A few years later, I found myself in Europe studying for my master's degree at the London School of Economics. London was a huge change from New York City. I noticed that my German, Italian, and French classmates at school cooked a lot—dinner was always made from scratch at home, our kitchen constantly in use. People seemed to place a lot of value on fresh, organic, sustainable ingredients and enjoying meals with friends over good conversation, wine, and delicious dishes. Furthermore, they were happy, healthy, and didn't deal much with weight issues. I wanted to have this kind of relationship with food! Suddenly I found myself eating a lot differently—and my energy returned. My skin brightened, my mind was sharper. I got sick less and could work out longer. I lost weight and didn't have to sacrifice for it. Eating healthily soon became nothing short of bliss to me. I had finally awakened to the fact that food connected directly with our wellness and that eating like this was delectable, fun, and simple.

I became so enamored with healthy food and where our food comes from that upon returning to the United States, I made a big decision. Instead of working on Wall Street, I changed course altogether and plunged myself into the world of food, health, and public policy. I did a remote internship at the Institute for Agriculture and Trade Policy, and coauthored a paper on the dangers of high-fructose corn syrup. I also began writing for a nonprofit organization called the Eat Well Guide. I then took an even bigger leap and enrolled in a professional chef training program at the acclaimed Natural Gourmet Institute in New York City—one of our nation's foremost culinary schools for health-supportive cooking. After the first day, I fell deeply in love. Cooking was the artistic expression I had been after for so many years. Paired with the education on whole and healthy food, I knew I had the perfect recipe for a lifelong relationship with healthy eating.

But I didn't stop there! Oh, no. I got certified as a personal trainer, and with the combination of food, cooking, and exercise knowledge, I launched a healthy lifestyle

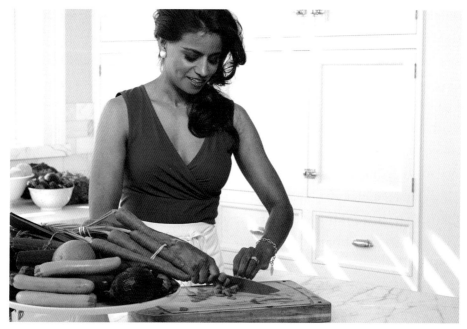

The tip of your knife has the power to release vibrant WAMP flavors

consulting practice in New York City. I started teaching others the joys of healthy foods and healthy living. For the next few years, my bustling practice brought me people from all walks of life, from college students to stay-at-home moms, to financial executives to artists. I taught each client how he or she could change her day-to-day food choices with little sacrifice and boatloads of pleasure. My clients were thrilled with their progress— and incredulous! A simple yet powerful plan finally helped them eat healthier with little sacrifice and minimal rules.

What I know—and what you're going to learn in your Resets—is that most people's problems with healthy eating can be solved with just two lessons: (1) understanding what healthy, whole foods *really* are, and (2) experiencing their taste by cooking simple, tasty recipes in your own kitchen. With these two skill sets, practically anyone can get on the path to eating healthily for good.

The 3-Day Reset program is simple but revolutionary. Most food advice comes from registered dieticians and nutritionists, but with my expertise in business, cooking, and health research, I bring something very new to the table. I approach it with practicality and enjoyment in mind. My plan empowers *people*, not their medical practitioners. In my opinion, healthy eating is supposed to come as naturally as brushing your teeth and taking a shower—in theory, we shouldn't need to be seeking advice on how to do it from anyone else. This is probably why my work has been so well received by companies like Whole Foods Market, where I teach classes—this program puts the power in your hands, and all that money you'll save on counseling sessions or expensive diet plans can be put toward healthy food, with plenty left over.

My life is just as nonstop as yours. I am a new mom to a beautiful girl named Valentina, work full-time as a businesswoman, and try my best to juggle career and family. Yet I don't compromise my health by eating the unhealthy, processed food that surrounds us. I've got the knowledge and the know-how that makes eating well an easy, delicious part of my every day. You will too.

What My Clients Say About 3DR

Enough from me—let's hear how my clients and students have embraced these Resets. My clients come from various walks of life, from academics to Silicon Valley CEOs. The majority of my private clients are men and women who embody the "work hard, play hard" lifestyle. Many of them hold executive-level positions on Wall Street and in other areas of finance and venture capital. They also work in industries such as media, journalism, and marketing. And still others, especially my female clientele, are entrepreneurs who have chosen to leave the MBA-saturated, corporate, nine-to-five world to build their own small businesses.

Regardless of their chosen paths in life, one thing is clear about all of the individuals who work with me: They are passionate about changing their lives through healthy eating. My clients want to be healthier, and want to learn how to be in better control of their food choices, regardless of their hectic lifestyles.

One client of mine had been working with a personal coach for two years, working toward reaching his career goals. He's a forty-something Wall Street executive, married with two young kids, and he realized that healthy eating was in fact a key piece of his career and life success. But he didn't know where to start. His career coach didn't know a lot about healthy foods or how to cook them, so he couldn't get guidance there. He also didn't have the time, patience, or willingness to change his entire eating routine. He was changing jobs, and that, along with his family, was a top priority. He also loved food and didn't want to sacrifice too much. After learning about me on the Internet and through my articles, he contacted me and we began to work on several Resets together. After just three weeks, he said he had learned and experienced more about healthy food than he had ever thought possible, and that the whole experience was surprisingly enjoyable and so much better than other "detox" or "cleanse" programs he had tried in the past:

> "When I did a juice cleanse, every day I was hoping it would end—it was really an ordeal. But the things that Pooja recommends are easy to do, they don't require sacrifice, and I learned a lot about new flavors—it was exciting."
>
> **—Kevin, Wall Street professional**

Here's another great example of the success of the The 3-Day Reset plan. Last year, a female college student came to me to help her lose some weight and find a "glow" to her skin and appearance. She knew little to nothing about whole foods or simple home cooking, and was curious to learn how to navigate her food choices (especially since she was on a budget) in the midst of all the dormitory-prepared meals and heavily processed, street-cart food. After undergoing a series of Resets, she began to completely rethink how she defined "healthy food," and she not only felt cleaner and leaner, but much more in control of the foods that surrounded her. For the first time, she became mindful in deciding what to place on her plate, and paused before purchases at the cafeteria and bodega. She actively sought out healthier, whole food–based brands and varieties of foods and started to cook for the first time in years! She saw her journey as a revolutionary, empowering experience that didn't cost her any hardship—it was all just a lot of fun. To this day, she continues to weave simple home cooking into her weekly schedule and has shed what she called "baby fat" without doing anything more than eating delicious, nourishing, whole food.

> "The Resets work for me because they aren't intimidating. Most 'cleanses' have all these built-in expectations—a lot of which are projected by the

individual. There is this pressure to do the cleanse right, or do it all the way, not make any mistakes. With The 3-Day Reset, all of that pressure evaporates. These are small, easy changes that you make over three days. That's it. With just these small changes, you can feel an amazing difference.

My personal best experience has been with the 3-Day Wheat Reset. When I'm feeling tired or overworked, I know I can get back on track just by eliminating wheat and wheat products. That's why it's called a 'Reset': It takes you back to a clean square one. What you take with you is an awareness and understanding of how certain foods affect your body. What's exciting about the Resets is that you don't know how your body responds to certain foods if you have them every day. I remember the first time I did the Wheat Reset. I called my mother and said: 'I didn't even realize how tired I was until I was awake!' That's why these Resets are so powerful, and so crucial."

—Jane, student, New York University

My clients tell me over and over that they have experienced sustainable, life-changing, and eye-opening epiphanies. They've told me how they couldn't believe how much a seventy-two-hour process could change their food decisions—forever. They've noticed how rethinking their approach to food choices has made them feel more relaxed, more in control, and more empowered with what they choose to put in their bodies. They've taken on active roles instead of passive ones, and that always feels good.

Yet, most important of all is that what I tend to hear the most is that after the Resets, my clients are blown away by the flavors they are suddenly experiencing! They love the "wow" factor that comes with craving wholesome food. I've never once heard the word "compromise" from anyone I've trained. And that, to me, is the true essence and brilliance of The 3-Day Reset! You'll *want* this. You'll *enjoy* this. And you're ready for it.

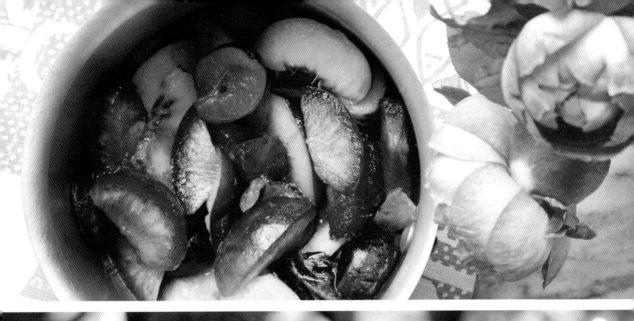

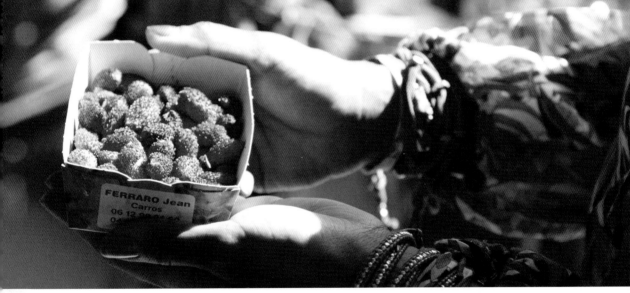

FERRARO Jean
Carros
06 12

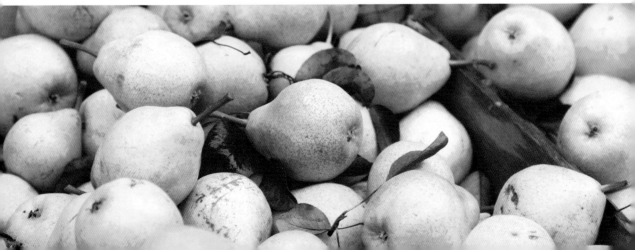

What Is a RESET?

Every chapter in this book is a unique Reset. There are ten Resets altogether:

- The first three Resets are for the most common ingredients that surround us every day: sugar, salt, and wheat.

- The next four Resets are for popular foods and drinks: chocolate, yogurt, chicken, and beverages.

- The last Resets are common meals and dishes: breakfast, salads, and take-out dinners.

Why do I focus only on these ten categories? Because the world of food is too complicated to attack it all at once.

Just think about it: If we were to examine each and every food product available to us individually, we'd be sitting here for years! The average size of a supermarket is 40,000 square feet, and on those endless aisles are some 40,000 products, all with different ingredient lists. There are also hundreds of books, magazine articles, and programs all focusing on the "right" foods to eat. How do we sort through this complicated heap of information on a subject as vast as "food"?

The answer: Keep. It. Simple. Ten Resets, enjoyed three days at a time, is all it takes to make impactful, lifelong changes. What you'll find is that you will easily be able to take what you will learn and experience from just these ten categories and apply it to countless more food products, dishes, recipes, and restaurant menus. Think of these ten 3-Day Resets as all you need to get on the path to restoring your cravings for healthy foods for life.

> There are hundreds of diet books, magazine articles, and programs all focusing on the "right" foods to eat. How do we sort through this complicated heap of information on a subject as vast as food?

What You'll Learn

From vegan cupcakes to gluten-free bread, trying to figure out what's healthy and what's not is nothing short of a Herculean task. Are cookies healthy because they're "USDA certified organic"? No, they're still full of refined sugar. Are all drinks with antioxidant-rich pomegranate and blueberries healthy? Nope, not if they're full of flavorings and preservatives. What about soy? Well, that depends on what form it's in and how it was made.

It's completely understandable that identifying what's healthy and what's not is a tall order for the average person. Our food has become so altered and so far removed from its source by the food industry, that we don't even know its real origins. Most of us have no idea how foods are made. Our food has become so incredibly processed by food companies that even the foods we think are healthy are engineered to the hilt—what I call "fake healthy." Nearly 70 percent of what we eat comes in packages, bottles, or boxes, toting nutrition labels, various health claims, and heavy doses of marketing—much of it "fake healthy" food.

In the first part of each of the Resets that follow, you'll get the chance to learn a unique set of skills that cut through the fog and allow you to pinpoint the best foods for you with clarity and ease, essentially resetting how you know food. You'll be learning about the provenance, history, and facts behind some of the most everyday, run-of-the-mill foods like yogurt and cereal because in order to accurately assess food, you have to look at the big picture and get to know it on a deeper level. In the end, you'll have the tools to identify truly healthy food when you see it, and spot the "fake healthy" food that's trying to trick you.

What You'll Experience

However, it's not enough to reset how you know food; you've also got to touch it, smell it, taste it, work with it, and see it. In other words, you've also got to reset how you experience food. It's like learning how to swim. You can read all about how the breaststroke works in books and watch many instructional videos, but unless you yourself dive into the pool and try it, you'll never stay afloat. It's the same thing with healthy eating. In order to restore our cravings for healthy foods, we need to take what we learn and put it into practice. In the words of Nike, we need to "just do it." That's why the second part of each Reset in this book asks you to start cooking and take small steps to raise your awareness of the food that surrounds you in your daily life. This section of a Reset is denoted by the motto "Ready, Set, Reset." It's followed by a set of simple instructions, a grocery list, and recipes to be made and enjoyed over a short three-day period.

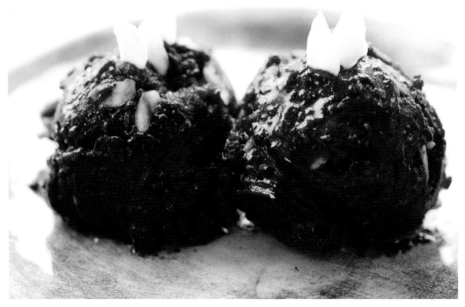

Strawberry & blackberry almond sorbet

After years of studying, teaching, and consulting on healthy, whole foods, I learned a valuable lesson: It's impossible to make healthy eating a permanent part of your lifestyle without enjoying it. In other words, we can't eat healthily unless we love eating healthily. Eating healthily shouldn't be hard. In fact, that's how humans work. We're chemically hardwired to be drawn to foods that make us feel pleasure—foods that taste good. It's not enough that our brains tell us what's healthy; our taste buds have to comply!

Luckily, you don't have to be fancy chef or even a stellar home cook to make nourishing food taste great. I designed these recipes to be short, easy, and manageable to even the most novice of cooks. We're not talking about complicated, time-suck cooking here. If you're worried you can't cook because you have a hard time dicing an onion or because you know you haven't turned on your oven in over a year, no need to despair! 3DR is a game changer because it's meant to make cooking healthy food easy.

In every Reset, you'll be discovering, exploring, and tasting—using all of your senses. You'll get an inside look at how exquisite flavor resides at the tip of your knife and cutting board. Delicious! You'll learn that seasoning food isn't just about butter and salt—it's about freshness, mixing and balancing flavors like savory, sweet, sour, bitter, and umami. It's about herbs, spices, diversity of ingredients, and the use of citrus, proper technique, aroma, and many other powerful factors. Some of the top chefs in the world know this, and now you can too. All of it will be a fiesta for your senses!

When I did a demo of my healthy summer salad recipes on WGN-TV, I remember the anchor telling me after the segment how surprised she was that the dish had so much flavor and it was so easy to make—she was amazed! When sharing my recipes, I've gotten this kind of response too many times to count. I can't tell you how many people have said, "Wow, Pooja, your food tastes amazing! I can't believe it's healthy and easy! Even *I* can do this!"

The secret is simple: Whole and minimally processed foods—healthy foods—and the dishes that can be created utilizing them are flavor superstars. Things like cacao, green tea, and authentically made yogurt have unique flavor profiles in and of themselves, and when combined with other simple, fresh ingredients to create specific recipes, the results are dishes that will blow your taste buds away.

Truth be told, in our current food environment—where most food prepared by others is unhealthy and processed—cooking is one of the only ways to ensure you can

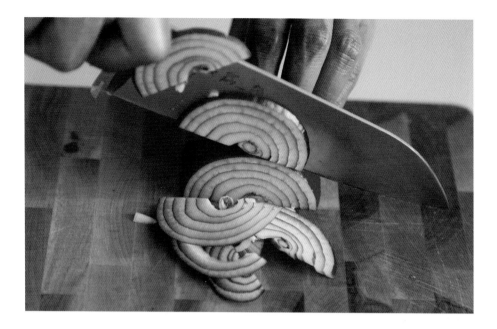

eat healthily. Cooking is your key to the castle. So take pride in it, even though you may be doing it for just three short days. When it comes to getting intimate with food, there's nothing more powerful than making it with your own two hands. If we're going to fix our problems with our modern diet, we need to roll up our sleeves, get out our cutting boards, and get to choppin'. There's no way around it: We've got to do in order to make change.

Why Three Days?

I created a Reset to last just seventy-two hours. Three days is the perfect timeframe to try something new and stick to it. You can do anything for just three days! And then, at the end of the Reset, you'll have become so immersed in a new way of eating that you won't be able to go back to the way you ate before. Seventy-two hours is all it takes!

Three days isn't very long, but it's still plenty long enough. And thank goodness for that. Let's face it: If I asked you to stop cold turkey eating a certain favorite food of yours, like bagels, for example, for twenty-one days, that's probably gonna be tough. You might feel pressure to never stray, and guilty if you do. That's a motivation killer, and why so many diets fail. But three days is easily achievable! It's a long weekend, or half a work-week. It'll go by in a blink—a delicious, empowering blink.

> Think of each 3-Day Reset as an amazing yoga retreat or once-in-a-lifetime, seventy-two-hour outdoor adventure. After you're done, you're guaranteed to come away inspired, renewed, and changed.

I found that three days is also the right amount of time to explore a wide range of flavors and variations of a healthy food or meal. It's also enough time to have an effect on your body. You'll a feel a difference in your mouth and your energy. That's because it takes, on average, a maximum of three days for us to fully digest and excrete the foods we eat. So if you go three days without refined sugar, for example, your body will likely feel a difference, especially since during those three days, you'll be fueling it with better, more nourishing foods.

The Results:
What You Can Expect From Doing a Reset

Success is individual, and this book is designed to allow everyone to succeed. Whether you're focused on just one or two Resets or all ten, by reading the Resets and taking action for three days at a time, you will successfully overhaul your understanding of food in a way that will change the way you choose, buy, make, and enjoy it for the rest of your life—ultimately restoring you to your natural cravings for healthy foods.

The more Resets you do, the more amazing the rewards. These Resets represent an enormous portion of what we eat every day, and by building on past Resets with new Resets, you will be putting yourself on the right path to making healthy eating automatic and long-term. That's how powerful this book can be! You'll realize that you'll be hard-pressed to go back to your old ways of interacting with food. You'll find that you'll be more attracted to the right kinds of foods and your taste buds will have had the opportunity to fall in love with the kinds of ingredients and dishes that love them back.

With 3DR, you'll change what you put in your body forever.

The Power
OF WAMP!

Read a chapter, cook a bit, and eat what you've made all over a three-day period, and *bam*! You're on your way to restoring your cravings for healthy foods. That's the CliffsNotes version of what this book asks of you. In the chapters that follow, we're going to be learning a lot about what we're eating, and we're going to start munching less on processed foods and more on what I call WAMP foods. It all begins with these two simple principles:

Processed Foods = Bad
<u>W</u>hole <u>a</u>nd <u>M</u>inimally <u>P</u>rocessed Foods (WAMP) = Good

WAMP is key to 3DR. It offers a bulletproof definition of healthy food—a definition that supersedes the terms "organic," "natural," and "local."

WAMP It Up

The idea that eating whole foods is good and processed foods is bad may seem self-evident, but it's not as obvious as you might think. In fact, pinpointing WAMP foods isn't simple. Processed foods can be sneaky and disguise themselves as healthy foods without our noticing.

For example, we all know that chips, fries, and doughnuts are processed junk-type foods—that's obvious. But what about bagels, cereal, and yogurt? Maybe not—it all depends on the ingredients that make them what they are. Most bagels are full of refined, processed wheat, and mainstream cereals are stuffed with processed sugar—they're certainly not WAMP foods. The fact is there isn't a standard, regulated definition of the words "whole" or "minimally processed." You'll need to learn what makes a food WAMP and what doesn't because labels on packages won't tell you.

Luckily, there are a few key attributes that flag a food as WAMP.

Direct From Mother Nature

Let's start by defining "whole foods." Whole foods are foods that come directly from Mother Nature, period. What this means is that these foods look pretty much the same whether you find them at a grocery store or on a farm. Whole foods, for the most part, come from the plant, animal, or fungi kingdoms. Carrots, whole chickens, mushrooms—they're all considered "whole."

Take cinnamon sticks, for example. They're bark, from plants, and we find them essentially as is, direct from nature. Same with coconuts, apples, lettuce, and hundreds of other foods. Once those foods are processed, though, they lose their nutrient power and goodness—they're no longer WAMP.

The key here is that whole foods are *unaltered* from the way you'd find them in the wild.

Minimally Touched by the Human Hand

With "minimally processed foods," a little common sense goes a long way. For example, minor alteration by the human hand is necessary for some whole foods to be stored, shipped, preserved, and consumed. Some fish are smoked to prevent them from going bad. Whole chickens are skinned, deboned, and fit into convenient packages for

✔ Whole Food	✔ Minimally Processed Food
Almonds	Unsweetened Almond Milk
Raw Cacao Pod	85% Cacao Dark Chocolate
Wheatberries	Whole-Wheat Pasta
Orange	Fresh-Squeezed Orange Juice
Whole Chicken	Skinned, Deboned, and Marinated Chicken Breast
Peanuts	Raw Peanut Butter

us to pick up from the supermarket. In the preparation of chocolate, cacao beans need to be extracted from the pods they came in, fermented, and dried prior to consumption. Butter needs to be made by humans from the milk of animals. Juice needs to be squeezed out of a fresh orange in a similar way to how olive oil needs to be extracted from the olive.

All of these are great examples of minimally processed foods. We don't find them as is in nature, but they're changed only in small ways for us to better consume them.

With just a little common sense and some thinking about the origins of foods, knowing what's minimally processed becomes simple. Above is a chart that helps show how we transform whole foods into minimally processed foods.

Keep It Real

Another key attribute of WAMP foods is their deep-rooted connection to the history of food, culture, and ancient ways of cooking and eating. WAMP foods tend to be key ingredients in authentic recipes of traditional cuisines. For example, when our ancestors made some of the very first breads, they did so with WAMP ingredients: whole-wheat kernels crushed using millstones (minimally processed), unrefined sea salt, wild yeast (sourdough starter, not baker's yeast), and water. Same with yogurt: A traditional food

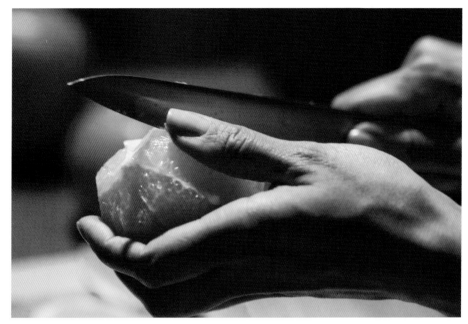

Oranges and their fresh-squeezed juices are wonderfully WAMP

of the Balkans, it was likely made from the milk of pasture-raised animals (goat, sheep, or cows) and wild bacteria (not a manufactured strain as is the case today in most of the Dannons and Yoplaits). Even the first pizzas were likely made using minimally processed flours, fresh herbs, fresh cheese from pasture-fed animals, handmade olive oil, and tomato sauce—nothing like the kind of pizza pies we eat at Pizza Hut. WAMP ingredients and dishes tend to be those that have been around for the longest—through generations. They're old school.

Super WAMP

Okay, so you must be thinking at this point, *Why aren't we talking about "organic" or "non-GMO"*? If WAMP foods are organic, local, sustainable, or otherwise produced in a healthier way for us and the planet (i.e., without pesticides, without antibiotics, without genetic modification, etc.), they're superior—or what I like to call "Super WAMP." An organic banana is a better WAMP food than a conventionally grown banana. Sustainably grown rice is a better WAMP food than genetically modified rice.

WAMP Tip-Offs

- WAMP foods are usually perishable: They won't last too long on that top shelf in your pantry.

- WAMP foods usually don't come with ingredient labels. If they do, they'll likely have fewer than five ingredients.

- WAMP foods rarely have ad budgets. You'll never see a commercial or advertisement for them.

- WAMP foods don't have "natural flavor" in their ingredient lists.

- If, after some basic investigating, you can't figure out where the food you're eating came from, it's probably not WAMP!

Eat Super WAMP foods when you can, especially when choosing foods from animal origins. Remember, though, that a food labeled "organic" doesn't make it WAMP. Doughnuts, table sugar, cookies, and potato chips can be "organic," but WAMP? Usually not.

The Science

Now we get to the part about why WAMP foods are the best foods for us, and why they're so "good." Science loves WAMP. Researchers agree that whole and minimally processed foods are more nutrient-dense than processed foods, and therefore healthier. WAMP foods contain more fiber, vitamins, minerals, phytochemicals, and so on—more of the disease- and cancer-fighting good stuff—than processed foods.

The case for WAMP foods is only getting stronger each year. Study after study reveals that these foods, especially plant-based WAMP foods, can help prevent certain cancers, diabetes, heart disease, and obesity.

The idea that the whole is better than the sum of its parts, a quality described as "synergy," takes WAMP foods to the major leagues. Scientists have realized that whole foods have a certain *je ne sais quoi* that foods made by humans don't, a characteristic that is best exemplified by what happens when you eat a whole carrot versus ingesting

"Natural" Doesn't Mean Much

Although the word "natural" seems honest and nurturing to most of us, truth be told, there is no official, regulated definition of the term. According to the FDA, the agency "has not developed a definition for use of the term natural or its derivatives."

However, in using the word "natural" to describe meat and poultry products, the USDA does regulate the term, requiring "these to be free of artificial colors, flavors, sweeteners, preservatives, and ingredients that do not occur naturally in the food. Natural meat and poultry must be minimally processed in a method that does not fundamentally alter the raw product. In addition, the label should explain the use of the term natural, e.g., "no artificial ingredients."

At the end of the day, the word "natural" doesn't guarantee us *anything* unless it's used to refer to meat and poultry products.

a pill that contains beta-carotene. You don't get the same benefits from the pill; eating the carrot is better.

Science has found that there's a special synergy among nutrients in whole foods that humans can't replicate. When we take a bite out of a carrot, hundreds of nutrients within that bite of carrot work together to ensure they function optimally—and provide us with the nourishment we're meant to have from that carrot.

It's for this same reason that taking fish-oil pills (a product of extracting and isolating oils from whole fish and then encapsulating them) doesn't give you as much benefit as eating fresh, whole fish; why drinking apple juice just isn't as healthy as munching on a whole apple; why enriched white bread isn't as nourishing as wheat berries.

The bottom line is that WAMP foods have a quality that trumps the duplicative powers of modern medicine and nutrition science. We know they're uniquely healthy, yet we can't figure out how. But we do know that WAMP foods are the true definition—the *par excellence*—of healthy food.

Common Sense

Common sense tells us there *must* be something good about whole and minimally processed foods too. WAMP foods have been nourishing our species, helping us survive and reproduce for millennia. Moreover, most WAMP foods have been around for thousands of years, whereas processed foods made their debut only in the last century. We're built to run on foods that didn't come from a lab or factory or off some conveyor belt.

Trusting Mother Nature seems smart. Sometimes, trusting our instincts and taking cues from human history can help us find the way, even when science can't give us all the answers.

The Flavor

Ready for the best news about WAMP? This food is t-a-s-t-y! And it's no wonder, since our species is biologically hardwired to find WAMP foods pleasurable. In fact, scientists have found that humans acquired a sense of taste to help them stay alive—edible, nourishing WAMP foods generally tasted sweet (signaling we may eat them) while poisonous foods tasted very bitter (signaling the opposite).

The sweet flavor of ripe summer strawberries is euphoric. Oysters are deliciously salty. Mushrooms have the perfect touch of umami. These kinds of foods give us incomparable pleasure. Composed of hundreds of flavor compounds with beautiful hues, tantalizing textures, and heavenly aromas, WAMP foods deliver on many levels. And in their freshest state (harvested at the peak of ripeness and used shortly thereafter), nothing can beat the multi-sensory experience we can obtain from them.

Similar to the special synergy in their nutrient value, WAMP foods are made up of complex combinations of chemicals that affect their taste and smell—combinations that humans have a hard time replicating as well. For example, the potent oils found in an orange peel contain a mind-boggling combination of over 200 chemicals alone. The distinct flavor of pure maple syrup cannot be reproduced, the science behind its flavor a secret of Mother Nature.

The fact that most WAMP foods originate from the earth's soil may also contribute to their spectacular flavor. Trace minerals, like chromium and manganese which transfer from the ground to plant foods like herbs and vegetables, are thought to impart intense flavor to these foods.

> Composed of hundreds of flavor compounds with beautiful hues, tantalizing textures, and heavenly aromas, WAMP foods deliver on so many levels.

WAMP foods hit all points in the spectrum of the five basic tastes: sweet, sour, salty, bitter, and umami. Pure honey and dried figs deliver sweet; fermented foods like yogurt allow for sour; minimally processed cheeses and other dairy products yield saltiness; greens like endive and escarole give us bitter; mushrooms and meat provide umami. WAMP foods hold all the flavors, textures, colors, and aromas we require to fall madly in love with them.

And when we combine WAMP foods with the art of simple cooking and ingredient mixing and matching—as we will do in the Resets that follow—*et voilà!* WAMP foods become unimaginably delectable, a dream come true for our taste buds! This is one of the main premises of this book: that healthy, whole-food meals have the potential to be unimaginably delicious.

WAMP vs. Diet Plans: No Contest

Over the last seventy years or so, hundreds of diet theories have come and gone with none of them accomplishing what they set out to do. For example, the seeds for the "low-fat, low-cholesterol" diet were sown back in the 1950s based on work done by a physiologist named Ancel Keys. Keys found that consuming high levels of fat leads to heart disease, a hypothesis first referred to as the "diet-heart hypothesis." By 1961, the American Heart Association had largely backed this work, which opened the door to the "low-fat" craze still somewhat active today. Yet despite all the decades of developing low-fat foods, Americans are still fat, and heart disease continues to be the leading cause of death in America.

The vegan diet—which is all the rage these days—isn't bulletproof either. Studies have shown that even when red meat is eliminated from the diet, you're still not "heart-attack proof."

The "low-carb" diet doesn't make any sense, as some of the most nutrient-dense foods on the planet are vegetables, fruits, and greens—all carbs.

And as far as the Atkins diet is concerned, plenty of renowned physicians have refuted its effectiveness, even going as far as calling it "disease promoting" and "clearly atherogenic" (promoting fatty plaque in the artery).

There's Nothing Natural About "Natural Flavoring"

Although we'd like to think of "natural" as wholesome and nourishing, unfortunately, when it comes to modern food marketing and flavoring, we can't. Although natural flavorings are made with ingredients derived from nature as opposed to synthetic ingredients, they're still made in high-tech laboratories by professional "flavorists" in white lab coats.

The FDA defines "natural flavoring" as "the essential oil, oleoresin, essence or extractive, protein hydrolysate, distillate, or any product of roasting, heating or enzymolysis, which contains the flavoring constituents derived from a spice, fruit or fruit juice, vegetable or vegetable juice, edible yeast, herb, bark, bud, root, leaf or similar plant material, meat, seafood, poultry, eggs, dairy products, or fermentation products thereof, whose significant function in food is flavoring rather than nutritional."

In other words, natural flavorings can come from things as obscure as "buchu leaves" and "angola weed." Moreover, if a natural flavoring reads as a "natural" strawberry flavoring, it doesn't mean that it came from a strawberry.

Staking a claim in the "best diet" arena is nothing short of a futile practice. Given the inability to scientifically control the hundreds of factors that play into our unique lifestyles and genetics, and the deep complexity of the human body, making a judgment call on which diet plan is perfect for the broad population is pretty much impossible.

Yet the one thing we do know is that foods in their least altered state—WAMP foods—are, hands down, better than processed foods, and when we start consuming these foods exclusively, we'll no doubt be a lot better off than we are now. It's just that simple. For many people, just the transition from processed to whole food can help reverse and stave off many ailments such as overweight, allergies, and chronic disease.

In this book what I'm claiming is that eating foods like these will give us our *best shot* at living a long, healthy, and happy life. By getting back to eating whole, traditional and ancient ingredients and foods, we'll make some serious strides with our health. And in this sense, eating WAMP foods is *indeed the best way to eat* for the vast majority of us.

A Closer Look at Processed Foods

Let's now turn our attention to processed food and why we shouldn't be eating it. Processed food is all food that's not WAMP. These days, 70 percent of our calories come from processed foods, most of which make up the 40,000 or so products you can find right now at your neighborhood supermarket.

Refined ingredients like white flour and corn syrup, and the foods they go into like canned soup and frozen dinners, are all processed. In fact, in 3DR I consider the terms "refined" and "processed" as interchangeable, as most refined foods require excessive alteration from their whole-food origins and most processed foods contain refined ingredients, particularly refined sugar, refined fat (i.e., oils), and refined salt, usually in combination. These substances are known to tempt our palates and lure us into eating more of them by loading them up with chemicals that tell our brains "this is good, eat me!" when we shouldn't and don't need to.

All artificial sweeteners are processed too—they're not found in nature. Processed foods are made in factories and laboratories and slapped with brand names from companies like Nestlé and Kraft. In fact, many of the same companies that make processed food are the same companies that make animal feed, dog food, and soap.

You can't make processed foods using grandma's recipe and your own two hands—they're foods that require serious engineering and high-tech genius.

Processed foods are also characterized by their use of additives. There are nearly 5,000 different kinds in our food supply—preservatives, colorings, flavorings, and fragrances. There are entire industries dedicated to creating fragrances and flavorings, from cinnamon to mint to lavender. Trained chemists known as "flavorists" at companies like Givaudan and International Flavors and Fragrances spend their entire careers in white lab coats engineering "artificial flavors" and "natural flavors" for companies like Coca-Cola and Unilever to use in their processed food and beverage products. Flavorists can make processed foods smell like chocolate without having anything to do with the cacao bean.

Ingredient lists of processed foods are uncannily unique, filled with items like guar gum, soybean oil, soy protein concentrate, natural flavoring, vitamin D2, riboflavin, and potassium chloride. There are so many strange sounding ingredients unique to processed foods that we could create a dictionary's worth.

The Work of Food Scientists

What's the function of processing? To make foods cheap; to make them taste a certain way; to make them easier to manufacture, ship, and store; to increase their shelf life (i.e., their expiration dates); to make them look better; to improve their texture; and, most importantly, to make them taste better because with all the dehydration, pasteurization, canning, irradiation, freezing, sterilization, and other feats of food-engineering wizardry that go into making processed food, their flavor is all but destroyed.

An entire field of work and study is dedicated to perfecting these functionalities. Food scientists garner degrees from prestigious institutions like Purdue University's Department of Food Science, where the food science curriculum is described as "an interdisciplinary field that applies the basic sciences, mathematics, and engineering to convert agricultural commodities into edible foods and beverages through various processing steps." These scientists spend their careers inventing new ways of improving processed foods and their ingredients at companies like Kellogg, Heinz, and Sara Lee. Food scientists have helped launch some of the most beloved processed-food brands in the history of the business, from Lunchables to Snackwells to Pop-Tarts.

Obviously, there are various grades of processed foods. For example, wheat. After wheat kernels are harvested, they're usually milled to make flour, which is then used to make breads and all sorts of baked goods. WAMP flour would be made from the simple grinding of wheat kernels by hand or stone mill. But a more highly processed flour might be made by removing the bran and germ of the wheat kernel ("refining") and then grinding or milling it mechanically at an industrialized mill—which would result in the same wheat flour we see today. This refined flour may then be used to make cookies for a brand-name company like Nabisco. The first flour required few steps, the second flour multiples more.

Flavorings

Flavorings, both natural and artificial, also play a role in food addiction. A *60 Minutes* exposé went behind the scenes of flavorings giant Givaudan in 2011 to find that flavorists there pride themselves on concocting flavorings that create cravings. So along with salt, sugar, and fat, flavorings in processed foods also boost their addictive qualities.

At right, we revisit our WAMP foods chart, except now we've added in an additional step where WAMP food is transformed into a processed food.

Processed foods don't contain the same amount of nutrients as WAMP foods—we know they're not as healthy. They don't contain as much fiber, minerals, or vitamins. And because they're devoid of that "synergy" quality that's inherent in whole foods, they can't deliver as much nourishment, even if they say "fortified" or "enriched."

Mother Nature didn't create processed foods—we did. And common sense tells us that because of this one simple fact, they're not perfectly designed for us. Another way to think about it is that, unlike WAMP foods, processed foods aren't vital to our survival. We can live quite happily—actually, extremely happily—without Cheerios, Eggo waffles, Red Bull, Tropicana Pure Premium, table sugar, and white flour.

Processed Food Is Addictive

Less than adequate in the health department, processed foods are bad in more ways than one. They do something very dangerous to our bodies—they exploit our biological weaknesses. By playing on our natural human susceptibilities, processed foods trick us into wanting to eat them even when we don't need to.

It works like this: If we backtrack some tens of thousands of years ago, our ancestors lived in a world that was characterized by scarcity. There wasn't enough food to go around—especially things like energy-boosting natural sugars (from fruits) and calorie-dense fats that were critical to our ability to survive and reproduce.

Living in this state in the natural world required signals to help us find these kinds

✔ Whole Food	✔ Minimally Processed Food	✘ Processed Food
Almonds	Unsweetened Almond Milk	Almond Joy Candy Bar
Raw Cacao Pod	85% Cacao Dark Chocolate	Chocolate Chip Muffin
Wheatberries	Whole-Wheat Pasta	White Bread
Orange	Fresh-Squeezed Orange Juice	Packaged Orange Fruit Drink
Whole Chicken	Homemade Chicken Soup	Frozen Chicken Tenders
Peanuts	Peanut Butter made of fresh peanuts and salt	Brand-name Peanut Butter with Additives and Preservatives

of foods. Since sugar and fat were hard to come by, they needed to stand out—and the way they did this was through their flavor. Both fruits and fatty foods (animal fat, animal milk, etc.) tasted delicious to our ancient ancestors (pleasing our palate was their signal), and thus they grew attracted to them. After all, if they didn't taste good, they'd have passed them up.

Over the course of thousands of years, these signals and have been imprinted into our neural circuitry through modifications to our genetic code. It's become automatic, hardwired inside us to want foods that are sweet, fatty, and even salty—especially foods that give us the most amount of each with the least amount of energy expended.

These days, our food environment looks shockingly different than it did 100,000 years ago. We no longer live in a world of food scarcity. Not only can we get our hands on fatty, sugary, and salty foods practically anytime of the day, we can get highly concentrated versions of them, thanks to the food-processing industry.

For example, we don't have to settle for the degree of pleasure derived from the *natural* sweetness found in an apple when we can get a supercharged version from the *concentrated* sweetness found in a candy bar made with highly refined table sugar.

We succumb to the candy bar because even though our food environment has evolved, we haven't. We're still wired to seek out the most pleasurable food with the least amount of work, no matter if it's less nourishing.

That's why we have a heck of a time freeing ourselves from the spell of frozen pasta dinners, caramel lattes, sodas, and french fries. These kinds of foods have been pinpointed as clinically "addictive," similar to drug addiction. Some psychologists now design programs to help treat what they refer to as "food addictions."

Processed Food Desensitizes Our Taste Buds

Processed foods are dangerous in a third, highly destructive way: They alter our taste buds, preventing them from finding WAMP food delicious. In other words, they change the sensitivity of our taste buds so we find less pleasure in healthy foods than we should.

The way it works makes perfect sense. Say your friend enjoys dessert, and almost every day she finishes dinner with a cookie. Now say she was forced to swap out her cookie for a piece of fruit, like a mango or a banana. Even though these fruits have some of the highest sugar content of all foods found in nature, she'd probably think they're not sweet enough in comparison to her regular cookie, and she wouldn't be as happy.

Now say we do a similar thing to another person who lives in a rural village somewhere in Thailand where access to processed cookies, and food in general, is limited. Say you gave this person the same pieces of mango or banana after dinner. He would likely find them very sweet—even blissfully sweet!

The difference in satisfaction can be attributed to the sensitivity of each person's taste buds. In enjoying the processed sweetness of cookies for so long, your friend had been unknowingly barraged with an extreme amount of sweetness that, over time, changed the sensitivity level of her taste buds, essentially dulling them. That's why, in taking a bite of the fruit, the sweetness didn't register. In order for her to find the pleasure she's after, she now needs very potent levels of sweetness, like those she gets from cookies that are made with refined sugar.

Whereas in the case of the villager, since he had never been exposed to processed food, his taste buds were never corrupted and remained normally sensitive. That's why he found the fruits extremely sweet and yummy. His taste buds could sense the natural sweetness.

A similar compromise occurs when we expose ourselves to salt. Given that most packaged, prepared, and frozen foods are doused with refined salt, we're unknowingly bombarding our taste buds with a level of saltiness that's not available to us in nature. The result: Over time, our taste buds lose their natural sensitivities to foods that are naturally salty (milk, meat, dairy), and we end up thinking that unsalted food tastes terrible.

> Processed foods threaten our healthy eating habits in a highly destructive way: They change the sensitivity of our taste buds so we find less pleasure in healthy foods from Mother Nature than we normally should.

Moreover, peer-reviewed scientific studies have found that the sensitivity of our taste buds is also influenced by the foods we choose to eat: We tend to enjoy the foods we're used to consuming (processed foods), and don't like the foods we're not used to consuming (WAMP foods).

Desensitization via processed foods has been discussed by many scientists who note that the more our culture becomes acclimated to processed, refined foods—foods that define the modern Western diet—the more eating WAMP foods becomes an unsatisfying, unexciting experience.

Now, let's get back to the simple principles we stated at the start of this chapter:

Processed Foods = Bad

Whole and Minimally Processed Foods (WAMP) = Good

The rationale behind this is now more than obvious. WAMP foods are healthier than processed foods, and full of fabulous flavor—they're "good." Processed foods are not as healthy and leave us addicted and our taste buds desensitized—they're "bad." If we eat more WAMP and less Processed we will restore our natural cravings for healthy food. Let's begin!

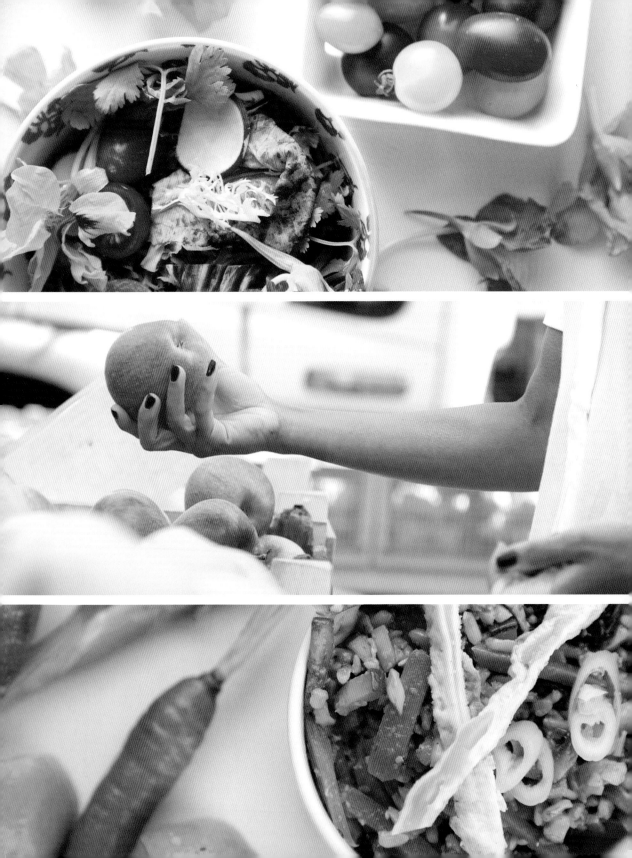

GETTING
STARTED

This book is all about you! It's been designed to support you and empower you in your goal of making healthy eating a permanent, delicious part of your life. And in that vein, it gives you the freedom to choose how you want to use these Resets in a way that's best for *you*. Here is some guidance to help you maximize your 3DR experience:

1. Start with the big guns.

The first three Resets—Sugar, Wheat, and Salt—are critical. You'll find these three ingredients in almost everything you eat on a daily basis. For that reason alone, it's a great idea to do the first three Resets first, and then continue on with the others.

2. Follow your inspiration.

You can easily flip open the book, find a Reset you're excited about, and jump in. Then, when you finish, you can choose another, then another. In other words, you can go in any order you choose. If you're eager to change how you eat breakfast, for example, start with the Breakfast Reset. If you've got a killer soda addiction you want to kick, start with the Beverage Reset. Love chocolate (and want an excuse to eat it)? Start with the Chocolate Reset. Again, totally up to you!

The only caveat is that you *must* read the chapters titled What is a Reset? and The Power of WAMP first, as they introduce you to the concept of a 3-Day Reset and WAMP—both integral to properly experiencing every Reset that follows. They lay the foundation for the entire 3DR program.

You must also review the 80/20 Rule, which is described below.

Tips

Now, for some tips!

- Choose the three days for each Reset wisely. For some Resets, you may feel you need to have more free time to focus on and enjoy them properly, and you'll want to do them over a weekend. Other Resets might be influenced by your weekday life—are you drinking too much soda or sugary drinks at work? Those are better planned for Monday through Friday.

- Cook ahead of time. If cooking the recipes in the Reset isn't feasible during the three days, cook and store the food before you begin the Reset. Then, when you're finished doing the Resets, put this book on your cookbook shelf so you can enjoy the recipes forever!

- If you love the recipes in this book, you can find more on my website, as well as videos in which I cook these recipes.

- Note the 80/20 Rule. At the end of each Reset, you'll notice the "After the Reset" section and mention of the "80/20 Rule." This rule is all about practicality. After you have finished the three days, you shouldn't feel obligated to eat *exactly* the same way going forward—it may be too extreme for you. Instead, shoot for the 80/20 Rule: 80 percent of the time you eat in accordance to the principles of the Reset and

20 percent of the time you don't (your wiggle room). This is the way I've eaten for years, and it's easy and achievable!

- You might want to consider holidays and celebrations when planning your Resets. For some, this is a perfect time to delve into a Reset journey because you have time off work and more energy to commit. For others, these days are more of an opportunity to let go completely and follow no rules at all. Based on your lifestyle, choose a path that works best for you. But whatever you choose, make sure to give it your all. It's only three days of your life!

- Keep in mind that with the Sugar, Wheat, and Beverage Resets, some people may experience mild withdrawal symptoms from the elimination of processed sweetness, caffeine, and processed carbohydrate from their diet. Slight headaches and lethargy are common and natural. It just means your body is adjusting from processed foods and excreting toxicity.

- Keep in mind that most recipes in this book have been developed to serve four people and the majority take thirty minutes or less. If you plan to cook for yourself and share the leftovers with friends or family on the same night, simply follow the recipe. But if you are cooking for one, I would recommend halving the recipe and storing the remainder for the next day or another time of day.

- Consider doing a Reset with a friend who has goals similar to yours. It's much more fun that way! Coordinate and share information, your thoughts, and what you experience. The more information sharing the merrier, and the more effective your Reset will be!

- Social media is also a useful tool for 3DR. As you embark on your three days, consider sharing the announcement of your excursions, daily epiphanies, and shifting food desires with friends, family, and your online community. Take pictures of your food and upload them to Facebook or Twitter. Use the hash tag #3DAYRESET to find others who are resetting alongside you. Blog about your experience. Boast about your new skills in the kitchen and with healthy food. Sometimes, sharing your journey with others makes it more inspiring and effective because others can help root for you and give you encouragement when you need it!

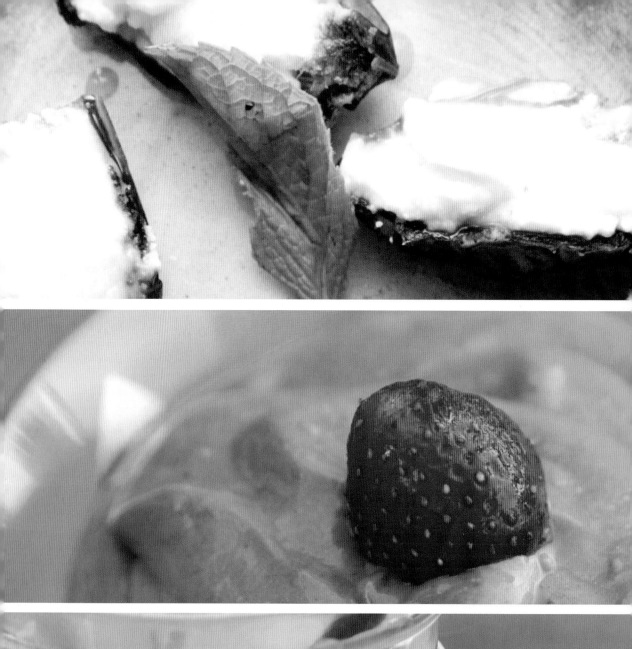
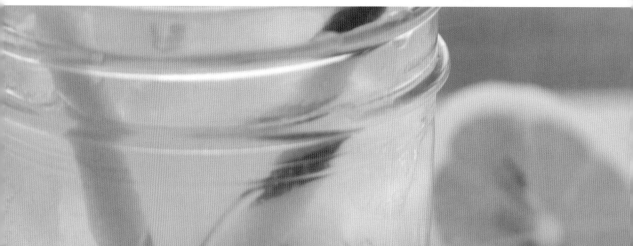

Sugar
RESET

Sweet stuff *rocks*. To many of us, sugary foods are as good as it gets—more tempting than sour, more satisfying than spicy, more comforting than salty. This makes sense since we're programmed to like sweet things from the moment we're born—one of the reasons why we enjoy our mother's sweet breast milk as babies.

The problem is, the majority of sweetness we're now eating doesn't suit our biology. Instead of satisfying our sweet tooth with things like ripe summer berries, dried figs, grapes, and raw honey (all WAMP foods), we're drowning ourselves with processed table sugar and corn syrup.

And it's everywhere. Processed sugar has managed to tiptoe its way into almost all kinds of foods without our noticing. It is a main ingredient in peanut butters, salad dressings, marinades, barbecue sauces, sports drinks, frozen pizza, and crackers. Even savory foods, like breads, pasta sauce, and chicken broth, are laden with processed sugars. Sadly, it's fair to say that sugar is the lifeblood of the food industry.

Sugar goes down like water, and we're consuming it with reckless abandon. According to the USDA, the average American eats about twenty-two teaspoons of sugar, or about 13 percent of our total calories, *each and every day*. Okay, let's think about this for a second: That's like opening up your kitchen silverware drawer, grabbing a teaspoon, jamming it into your sugar bowl, and sticking it straight inside your mouth twenty-two times a day.

It doesn't help that sugar is notoriously difficult to detect in foods. Not only is there no distinct line item for "added sugars" on the nutrition-facts panel of your food's label, but sugar also masquerades under a long and complicated list of aliases that would make even Jason Bourne weep with jealousy. "Dextrose," "fructose," "cane juice," and "maltose" all mean that sugar has been added to your food. Same with "invert sugar," "corn-syrup solids," and "lactose."

> According to the USDA, the average American eats about twenty-two teaspoons of sugar, or about 13 percent of our total calories, *each and every day.*

Apart from the obvious health consequences that arise from consuming too much processed sugar—like diabetes, weight gain, obesity, and hypertension—eating sugar may very well be the single biggest impediment to falling in love with healthy food. As we learned in The Power of WAMP, processed sugar exploits our innate biological weaknesses, lulling us into addiction and desensitizing our taste buds to the point that we can no longer find deliciousness in the kind of food that wants to love us back. When we become accustomed to processed sugar, suddenly, sweet WAMP foods become nothing short of sacrifices. A bowl of oats with cinnamon and banana pales in comparison to a vanilla-glazed scone from Starbucks or a bowl of Froot Loops. Even the best loose-leaf tea no longer tastes good without an extra sugar packet or two.

But we can—right now—slam on the brakes and put this train in reverse. All we have to do is reset our relationship with sugar. We need to put an end to our sugar ignorance and off-kilter sweet palate and relearn sugar from the ground up. We also need the opportunity to experience what it's like not to have processed sugar in our lives, and give our taste buds the chance to be awakened and excited by the superior flavor that comes from WAMP sweetness.

Little Packets of Crystals:
What You Need To Know about Sugar

It's not as if Mother Nature didn't want us to enjoy the taste of sugar in our lives. Humans *need* sugars, actually. Sugars provides us with quick energy, especially in times of depletion. And in Eastern medicine, sweetness is thought to be vital for good health. We don't have to nix sugar from our lives entirely—we just have to eat *the right kind* of sugar.

Luckily for us, Mother Nature has provided us with foods that afford all the sweetness we need to survive. Sugar, a simple carbohydrate, is found in vegetables (in the form of glucose and sucrose), milk and dairy products (in the form of lactose), and even in grains. Ripe fruits contain the most sugars (primarily in the form of fructose), and that's why I refer to them as "nature's candy." Grapes, mangoes, and pineapples are some of the sweetest foods on Earth.

So is honey, mankind's original sweetener. Honey has been added to food as far back as the Neolithic period. Ancient Egyptians, Romans, Chinese, and Indians all used honey to coat fruits, flowers, and the seeds of plants. In fact, honey was the sweetener par excellence in much of the world until the end of the Middle Ages, although some countries used date or fig syrup, or grape juice.

Suffice it to say, Mother Nature never dreamed we'd have access to that sandlike, bright white stuff we now refer to as table sugar.

The story of granulated table sugar begins in ancient India, where sugarcane, a tropical grass four to twelve feet tall and one to two inches in diameter that looks similar to bamboo, grows wild. In its mature state, sugarcane is about 12-14 percent soluble sugars—the rest is fiber and water. Possibly as far back as 1200 BC, ancient Indians found that a sweet juice—opaque and dark green in color—could be extracted by chewing on these sugarcane stalks, what we now refer to as sugarcane juice. We read about it in the *Ramayana*, one of India's greatest epics, which tells of banquets with "tables laid with sweet things, syrup, canes to chew."

It wasn't until about seven centuries later that a "foray into the valley of the Indus" led Persians to discover these stalks. They called them "reeds" and were mesmerized by how they gave "honey without bees." Until then, there had been no other substance on Earth, apart from honey, that yielded such a sweet taste.

A few centuries later, the Gupta Dynasty (circa AD 500) uncovered a way—through boiling, drying, and cooling—to transform the juice into crystalline solids, which made it easier to transport. The Indians called this *sarkara*, the Greeks called it "solid honey," and later the Crusaders—after retrieving it during campaigns to the Holy Land—would refer to it as "sweet salt." From then on, it became so highly coveted—a "spice even rarer and more expensive than any other"—that from the Romans to the Arabs, everyone wanted to get their hands on it. By 1300, it was "worth its weight in silver."

From Cane to the Table

It didn't take long for sugar to go from WAMP to processed. Sugar makers found that by separating the molasses (a by-product of transforming the cane juice into syrup) from the crystal solids, a less moist, less brown, sweeter sugar would result. By the 1700s, this separation became de rigueur. Cane juice was heated and clarified, then condensed into a thick syrup in which sugar crystals formed. Molasses was pulled out by placing the product into an upright conical pot with a drain at the base. Over the course of days to weeks, the molasses would drip down, leaving behind a semihard, cone-shaped structure called a "sugarloaf" that required a hammer and "sugar nips" to reduce to edible pieces.

Engineering and food science took over from there. By the mid-1800s, a centrifugal machine was invented to mechanically separate sugar crystals from molasses, while vacuums and "multiple effect evaporators" helped extract any unwanted water, further concentrating the sucrose-laden crystals. And by 1860, sugar in the state that we now know it—tiny, granulated, white crystals—was invented at the Boston Sugar Refinery.

Sugar refining soon became an industry in and of itself, allowing for even more stripping of the sugar crystal by removing its outer coating and purifying it until it couldn't be purified any more through complicated processes like "phosphatation."

With these transformations, sugar became more "user friendly" and versatile. In its newly refined state, it was shelf stable and portable, and its extra sweet, granulated crystalline form the perfect complement to processed foods. It could now be added to foods to help preserve, enhance texture and color, and even to bulk up and ferment them.

Processing sugar leaves it nutrient-depleted. By extracting molasses from cane juice

> ## Terminology
>
> You'll notice that throughout *The 3-Day Reset*, I use the words "processed" and "refined" interchangeably for ingredients like sugar, wheat, and salt. Why? If an ingredient is refined, more often than not, it must have been altered extensively—either by man or by machine. So in this sense, it can no longer be a "WAMP" food and must be the opposite: a processed food.

and refining it to the nth degree, all the soluble fiber, vitamins, and minerals—a complex mix of nutrients inherent in WAMP sugarcane that work synergistically to make it an extremely health-promoting and low-glycemic food—are removed. All that remains are nutrient-empty calories.

The Knockoffs: Beets and Corn

But this is only half the story. A large portion of tiny, white granules of sugar don't even have origins in the "honey-bearing reed." Instead, they're from a white, conical-shaped root vegetable called the sugar beet.

In 1745 it was discovered that sugar beets contain a high degree of naturally occurring sucrose, similar to sugarcane. When Napoleon was faced with a British blockade of sugar imports in 1813, he called for the large-scale production of sugar from these types of beets in France. This involved a highly industrialized and chemically based process similar to the refining of sugar from cane, including steps such as diffusion, carbonation, and filtration. Like sugar from cane, sugar from beets is by no means WAMP. (Moreover almost all the sugar we get from sugar-beet production in the United States today is genetically modified.)

Corn also supplies us with processed sugar, namely in the forms of high-fructose corn syrup, dextrose, and glucose. Its story begins in the 1970s, when high-fructose corn syrup became a mainstream liquid sweetener and was added to soda as a substitute for sugar. Just like sugar from cane and beets, the production of HFCS depended on technology, but this time to an even greater extent. HFCS could only be made through a complicated scientific process that required the alteration of chemical bonds.

Today we're splitting our consumption of added sugar evenly among sugar cane, sugar beets, and corn-derived sweeteners. Below is a list of processed sugars you'll likely see on ingredient lists of some of your favorite foods. Note how many different names sugar masquerades under:

Common Processed Sugars Added to Our Foods
(From Sugarcane, Sugar Beets, and Corn)

- Brown sugar

- Corn sweetener

- Corn syrup

- Corn-syrup solids

- Demerara

- Evaporated cane juice

- Evaporated cane-juice solids

- Fruit-juice concentrates

- High-fructose corn syrup (HFCS)

- Invert sugar

- Malt sugar

- Sugar

- Sugar molecules ending in "ose" (dextrose, fructose, crystalline fructose, glucose, lactose, maltose, sucrose)

Sugar's Sneaky Loopholes

When things go incredibly awry with public health, the government usually likes to step in. This has happened in the case of cigarettes, alcohol, and illicit drugs, for instance. But when it comes to sugar, the U.S. government has failed us miserably.

First, the FDA makes it exceedingly difficult for us to figure out how much sugar we're really eating. A pesky loophole in the FDA's ingredient-labeling laws makes

---

Sugar Rush

Even supposedly "healthy" foods like protein powders, breakfast bars, bagels, oatmeal, and probiotic drinks are laced with sugar. Sugar lurks in some of the least common places. A mind-numbing 13 percent of our total calories come from added sugars alone—about 70 percent from food, the other 30 percent from drinks.

---

detecting the amount of added sugars in our foods nearly impossible. Try glancing at the "Sugars" line item underneath the "Carbohydrates" category on any nutrition label and you'll come up empty handed. That's because "Sugars" in this section accounts for *both* naturally occurring sugars (lactose in yogurt, fructose in fruit) as well as sugars that have been *added* to your food. So how do we find the number of grams of corn syrup, invert syrup, and cane-juice concentrate injected into the stuff we eat and drink? We don't.

Another source of confusion we might blame on the FDA is why so many forms of sugar turn up on a single ingredient list. Instead of just "sugar," it's common to see "corn syrup," "cane juice," and "fructose" all on the *same* ingredient list. As we now know, these are all forms of added sugar. Here's why: As food-labeling laws now stand, ingredients must be listed in order of how much they dominate the food contained in the package, with the weightiest ingredient listed first. Food companies know this and have found a way to game the system so sugar doesn't appear at the top of the list. By dividing "sugar" among several different names, they can list the sweeteners further down the list of ingredients. That way, when we're looking at labels, we don't see "sugar" screaming at us from the get go, tricking us into believing that sugar is playing a smaller role in the food we're eating.

Rid Yourself of Processed Sugar and Prepare for Big Time Flavor

As we learned in The Power of WAMP, processed sugar exploits our biological weaknesses for sweets. A slice of mango can't go toe-to-toe with a chocolate-chip cookie. Plain yogurt isn't as good as yogurt with sugar.

Luckily, resetting your relationship with sugar can level the playing field. Even better, it can be one of the most delectable experiences of your life. It works like this: When we start avoiding processed sugars, over time healthy foods start to taste like ambrosia, and unhealthy foods start to taste unpleasant.

Where Added Processed/Refined Sugar Lurks

Common Foods

- Barbeque sauce
- Ketchup
- Chicken broth/stock, veggie broth stock
- Chips
- Steak sauce
- Stuffing mix
- Sausage
- Bacon
- Pizza
- Fried chicken
- Mayonnaise
- Fish sticks
- Cured meats
- Canned soups
- Teriyaki sauce
- Pickled foods
- Pickled cucumbers
- Canned corn
- Bread sticks
- English muffins
- Pasta
- Crackers
- Biscuits
- Bread
- Croissants
- Instant flavored coffee
- Coffee creamers

"Health" Foods

- Salad dressing
- Granola bars
- Instant oatmeal
- Nut butters
- Sports drinks and bars
- Cream and dairy substitutes
- Milk alternatives (rice milk, soy milk, almond milk)
- Waffles
- Baby food
- Popcorn
- Applesauce
- Dried fruits
- Margarine
- Canned fruit and vegetables

Drinks

- Sodas
- Juice drinks
- Juice nectars
- Coffee drinks
- Iced teas

In 1822, American adults ate the amount of sugar equivalent to one can of soda every five days. Now, we consume that much *every seven hours.*

Delete processed sugars from your life, and the sensitivity in your taste buds will increase. Once dead, now they're alive! You'll find so much more satisfaction in food that you once found unsatisfying. Ripe raspberries will begin to taste crazy delicious. The sight of a luscious, freshly chopped cantaloupe will make your mouth water. Flavor in healthy food will become more complex, richer, and more decadent.

You may even find yourself transforming into a connoisseur of sweetness. The slice of banana bread you buy at the café may taste so unsuitably sweet you can't take more than a small nibble. Your favorite brand of mint-chip ice cream may taste harshly sweet. Cotton candy and M&M's might give you a headache. You may plead for the barista to put less sugar-doused Monin syrup in your hazelnut latte. You might still love your mom's pumpkin pie, but you'll prefer a less sugary, subtler version.

This has happened to me and my clients countless times, and the experience is truly liberating.

"After getting off processed sugary foods for a while based on Pooja's advice, I started sensing how sweet healthy foods are; things like nectarines and bananas are enough sweet for me—sometimes they're even too sweet. Foods that I ate and drank as a kid like Honey Bunches of Oats, Arizona Iced Tea, and Snapple are now way too sweet; I don't even like them. I drink a ton more water now."

—David, Environmental Analyst, NYC

More Joys of WAMP Sweetness

WAMP sugars are better for us—honey, fruit, and other minimally processed sugars like maple syrup and coconut palm sugar. Lucky for us, WAMP sweeteners are flavor superstars. They're poignant, powerful, and distinct, with serious character. They don't give you the harsh, single-note flavor that table sugar is known for. When you substitute processed sugars with foods like dates, honey, and mangoes, you open yourself up to experiencing better, more nuanced flavor.

As we learned in the chapter What Is a Reset?, the complexity of flavors in WAMP foods is nothing short of astounding. Pineapples have a deep, luscious tropical flavor with hints of both sweet and sour and a wondrous aroma; dates are moist with notes of caramel and honey.

> Lucky for us, WAMP sweeteners are flavor superstars—they're poignant, powerful, and distinct, with serious character. They don't give you the harsh, single-note flavor that table sugar is known for.

Maple syrup, for example, has a flavor chemistry so distinctive that even the most venerated flavor scientists can't replicate it. According to Cornell University researchers, maple syrup contains about 300 flavor compounds, such as furanone, strawberry furanone, and the sweet-smelling maltol, which provide its distinctive taste. Its flavor is described by expert sensory specialists, tasters, and scientists as having prominent notes of caramel, vanilla, honey, cereal, chocolate, and coffee. All those nutrients and minerals that aren't stripped away contribute to this unique flavor profile.

Other WAMP sweeteners also deliver better, healthier flavor. Raw honey, which contains more enzymes and micronutrients than conventionally made honey, is wildly aromatic with fruity, woody, and floral notes. Rapadura (also known as Sucanat), an unrefined, unbleached, whole, dried cane sugar, contains iron and is possibly the healthiest WAMP sweetener out there. Coconut palm sugar, made from the sap collected from coconut flower buds is also very high in vitamins and minerals. It tastes like rich caramel.

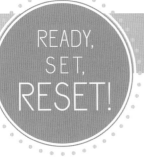

Ready to free yourself from processed sugar and start enjoying WAMP sweetness that's better for you? Now that we've been educated, it's crystal clear that our current relationship with sugar is beyond dysfunctional. This is our wake-up call.

It's time to reset sugar and empower ourselves. During this Reset, you'll see, touch, taste, and experience sugar anew. If you feel you're a sugar or dessert-loving person and need to have sweet foods every day, this Reset may be a bit more challenging for you. But remember, it's only seventy-two hours; you can do this!

Here's how it works. Once you have chosen three consecutive days for your Sugar Reset, you will spend those days *entirely without processed, refined sugars*. Any item that contains a processed sugar, whether a food or a drink, you'll avoid. This doesn't mean just those little white packages you use to sweeten your coffee, it means sugar in *anything*—in your restaurant dish, in the packaged crackers you like, in your vanilla soy latte, in the pasta sauces you use—everywhere.

Instructions

Here's how you'll do it:

- Examine ingredient lists on packaged foods.

- Ask your waiter about how your food was made—and your drink too!

- Check the list on page 48 that lists common forms of added sugars to help guide you while you investigate ingredient lists of the foods you want to buy.

- Be diligent and ask, ask, ask! If you're buying prepared food that doesn't announce its ingredients, investigate further or skip it.

While abstaining from processed sugar, you'll be exploring and discovering WAMP sweetness in a variety of glorious forms. Over the course of these three days, you'll have five kinds of sweetness to indulge in:

Choice 1: Ripe, Fresh or Dry Fruits

To help you manage your sweet tooth through this period, try sweet fruits such as mangoes, bananas, and pineapples, which have some of the highest sugar content of all fruits. Choose them very ripe, as in this state they are the sweetest. If you require even more sweetness, go for dried fruits like dates, figs, and raisins, which are much more sweet due to their concentrated levels of sugar. You can turn to these choices instead of your usual dessert after lunch or dinner, or as a substitute for your afternoon candy bar, cookies, or sugary snack. There's no need to go overboard here; eat only as much as you require to satisfy yourself. Take a balanced approach.

Choice 2: WAMP Sugar Crystals

As I mentioned earlier, a lot of processed sugar resides in what we sip, not what we chew. A lot of us start our day with coffee or tea with white sugar, so I'm including substitutes like Rapadura (also known as whole dried cane sugar or Sucanat), coconut-palm sugar, date sugar, or maple-sugar crystals to use instead. All of these can be found at your local health-food store and at most grocery stores. They're a bit pricier, but will last you a long time. You will also note that they taste more distinct, less sweet, and richer than white sugar. Substitute one-for-one for white sugar, but I recommend no more than one tablespoon per day. Bring these along with you to work if you like to sweeten your drinks on the job!

Choice 3: Maple Syrup

You may use maple syrup to sweeten your drinks too; just note that maple syrup has a very distinct and powerful flavor that may overwhelm other flavors. Again, substitute one-for-one for white sugar, but no more than one tablespoon per day. You may also eat a teaspoon of maple syrup straight if you need to satisfy a sweet craving over these three days. It tends to be sweeter than white sugar, so you'll only need a little!

Choice 4: Raw Honey

Raw honey has been used for thousands of years, cited in Greek, Islamic, and Vedic texts as a food of great healing abilities because of its powerful antimicrobial and antiseptic

> During this Reset, be a hawk when it comes to beverages. For example, most Starbucks coffee shops use soy milk with added sugar when making their hot coffee drinks, and most teas (both hot and iced) are made with simple syrups.

properties. It's been used topically to treat minor wounds and ingested to heal sore throats. The Greeks believe honey to have anti-aging properties. With more vitamins and minerals than white sugar, honey is more nutrient-rich. Substitute one-for-one for white sugar, but no more than one tablespoon (three teaspoons) per day. Like maple syrup, eat a teaspoon straight to ward off any sugar cravings while you undergo this Reset. I recommend raw honey because it contains more enzymes and nutrients than conventionally made honey.

Choice 5: Pooja's Recipes

Last, you may also choose to make the recipes at the end of this chapter. Two of them are intended as substitutes for sugary desserts. The third, a lemon-lime soda that's sweetened with maple syrup, is for those folks who depend on sodas or other sugary drinks every day. Plan to eat/drink no more than one to two individual servings of these per day.

TIPS & TOOLS for EACH DAY

Shutting white sugar down is no joke, but with some
tips and your substitute choices above, these next
three days will be nothing short of inspirational.

Day One

Good morning! This will be the first day you open your eyes to processed sugar. And
you'll likely be waking up to your first change of routine as you reach for your morning
joe. Instead of using white table sugar or brown sugar (which is simply white sugar with
molasses added back to coat it), try using an unrefined sugar crystal from Choice 2. If
you like to use cream, you'll want to make sure these are not sugar-laden as well. Most
coffee creamers have added refined sugars (e.g., Coffee-Mate).

If you're used to ordering your first beverage at a coffee shop, this is likely where
you'll also need to be on high alert. Make sure to ask the barista what's in the soy latte or
almond-milk cappuccino you're ordering. Most nationwide coffee chains, such as Starbucks, use nondairy with added sugar.

At breakfast, you'll want to look for more signs of sweetness. The almond milk you may
be using in your cereal likely has been sweetened with evaporated cane juice. Check the ingredient list. What's in your cereal? In your energy bar? Another tip: Unless a syrup is 100 percent
maple syrup, it's likely made of processed sugars, particularly high-fructose corn syrup.

At midday, you may notice the numerous sugar aliases in the ingredient list of your
granola bar or yogurt, or maybe in the crackers that you love to munch on every now and
then at your office desk.

Lunch is when you'll likely be doing a lot of asking. Be diligent at the salad or buffet
bar. Make sure the dressing isn't loaded with added sugars. If you can't find a list of ingredients, ask. If you usually frequent a restaurant or order take-out for lunch, you'll want
to be on the lookout for sugary marinades and sauces. Most sweet-and-sour, teriyaki, and
steak sauces have added sugars. So do pasta sauces and marinara. Ketchups too.

If you're finding that abstaining from your favorite juice drinks, bottled ice teas, or sodas is becoming hard, try sweetening sparkling water with maple syrup and a few squeezes of lemon or lime—a quick and easy WAMP beverage.

For your after-dinner dessert, try my recipes instead of your usual ice cream, cookie, or slice of pie. Savor and be mindful of every bite.

Over the course of this first day, try to zone in on differences in flavor, texture, and aroma you have discovered and experienced. How did the sweetness you had today compare with your usual sweet foods and drinks? How do you feel? Check in with yourself.

Day Two

Now that the first day is wrapped up, you'll have a better sense of what today's going to be like and you'll be more prepared. Congratulations! You're a third of the way there.

Today, see if you can trim down the amount of unrefined sugar crystals or honey or maple syrup you're using by just a tad and perhaps look to fuel your sugar needs more with fruit—humanity's original dessert.

Remember, this experience is not about banning sugar for the rest of your life or depriving you of delectable treats. This experience is about getting you *thinking*! The best way to open our eyes to how much processed sugar surrounds us is by going without it! These three days will give you the lay of the land and get you clued in more than anything else.

During your lunch break today or after work, if you end up going to the grocery store or bodega, take a few extra minutes to examine ingredient lists of some foods you buy on a regular basis. Look at things like snacks, juice drinks, frozen pizza, applesauce, and bread sticks. Is sugar embedded in the ingredient list? It's incredible what you will find.

Today, try cooking your dinner at home. This way you'll be certain no added sugars are in your meal.

You might also want to take time today to examine the bottled and packaged foods in your refrigerator, pantry, and freezer. What do you find? You'll realize that condiments are huge culprits. The ketchup and bottles of salad dressing that take up permanent real estate in your fridge all tend to contain processed sugars.

Day Three

Today, you'll want to keep up the pace and finish strong. You'll want to make sure you've tried as many of the above five WAMP substitutes so your senses can experience flavors that may have been foreign until now. How did dried dates taste to you? If you smear a dollop of honey and cheese onto your toast, what does that do to your taste buds?

If you had the chance to try any unrefined sugar crystals, what were your thoughts? You probably discovered that this form of sugar is a lot less sweet but has a ton of character and boldness that may have delighted your palate. If you couldn't try raw honey, maybe today is the day to do so.

On this third day, you may also have realized that you're craving that midday candy bar or Diet Coke a little less than yesterday, probably because you've given your taste buds a chance to free themselves from the attack of processed sweetness and regain a slight bit of their sensitivity. (If not, that's OK too; everyone's taste buds are different and operate on varying levels of sensitivity.)

You may also want to explore different fresh and dried fruits today. Great additions to the list above include ripe grapes, pears, and peaches as well as sundried tomatoes and dried bananas. Just make sure that when you're buying these, they haven't been coated with any sugars (cranberries are a prime example of this).

Make this last day count. If you haven't yet gone through your cabinets or pantry, take the time today to do so, and check out ingredient lists. You'll be surprised by what you uncover.

If you haven't had the chance to visit your local health-food store, try doing this today to check out what WAMP sweeteners are offered there. Maybe take some time to scour the Internet and do extra research of your own.

If you've been holding off on your favorite sugary desserts, don't give in. You only have twenty-four hours to go! Instead, try mixing and matching from the choices I've given you to create sweet recipes that make your mouth water—recipes that you know you'll love even after the Reset is over. Be creative. Be mindful. Be in the moment. Realize that you're empowering yourself!

Pantry Swap

White table sugar out, WAMP sweeteners in. Here is your new armory of healthier substitutes for table sugar:

- Whole cane sugar: unrefined, unbleached, also known by trade names "Rapadura" or "Sucanat." This is dried, unrefined sugar-cane juice and possibly the most nutrient-dense sweetener based on sugarcane there is. To make it, sugarcane is squeezed, filtered, dried, and ground (not separated at all). And no molasses is lost in the process, which means it's a lot healthier.

- Muscovado sugar: slightly more refined than whole cane sugar but retains some molasses and trace minerals depending on how it was milled.

- Coconut-palm sugar: farmers tap the coconut tree flower for its sweet nectar, similar to tapping a maple tree for syrup.

- Date sugar

- Maple sugar crystals

- 100% pure maple syrup

- Barley malt

- Brown rice syrup

- Molasses

- Organic honey (preferably raw)

- Jaggery or panela (traditional sugar blocks—harder to find)

Note: Brown, light brown, and dark brown sugar are not included as they're made by adding molasses to already refined white sugar crystals—a more processed sugar than whole-cane sugar, (which is brown because of the molasses that hasn't been removed). Demerara and turbinado sugars also tend to be more refined (less molasses) than those above. Keep in mind that the labeling of "healthy" sugars is complicated. Words like "natural," "raw," and "brown" are everywhere, but without standard, regulated definitions it's best to go with the list above and remember that the nutrient density (healthiness) of any sugar is based on how it was processed—period. One turbinado sugar may be less processed than another turbinado sugar, for example. So do your due diligence and be a smart shopper!

After the Reset

You made it! Congratulations on finishing this Reset.

With the combination of a sugar education and a seventy-two-hour sugar immersion, you've likely become extra aware of the amount of sugar you eat on a daily basis, where it's hidden and under what guises, and what it can do to your cravings and taste buds. Now you know the backstory of how processed sugars can manipulate you. You now know why it's hard to stop yourself from eating that next cookie, and you'll be better positioned to stop if you want to. And best of all, you've found WAMP alternatives.

After this Reset, you should have a completely new understanding of just how much sugar is added to the foods we eat. You're likely shocked that some of the foods you considered sugar-free, aren't. These revelations may prompt you to make some serious changes in your life. You may decide to switch the cereal and yogurt brands you've been devoted to for years, or change up your drink choices, or what you usually order for lunch.

> Take a few extra minutes to examine ingredient lists of some foods you know you buy on a regular basis. Was sugar imbedded in the list? It's incredible what you may find.

And because of the wondrous flavors you've had the chance to discover, you're now in a position to take control of your choices and fight back against the food industry. You know that figs and honey can satisfy you at times when you may have thought only sugar cookies could. You have more tools, more skills, and more knowledge.

And depending on the sensitivity of your taste buds before you started, you may have realized that, after this three-day period, foods that you once thought weren't so sweet (like granola bars and crackers) suddenly seem overly sweet. You may also have found that foods you didn't like as much, like fruits, taste a lot better than you remember.

As you go forward with your life and eating routine, you'll likely want to stick to my 80/20 Rule, which is outlined in the chapter Getting Started. There's no need to go rogue and stop eating processed sugar 100 percent of the time. There'll be birthday parties, bat mitzvahs, office events, and times when you just want to curl up in bed with some hot chocolate and a movie. These are all part of that 20 percent you'd do

YOUR SUGAR RESET GROCERY LIST

- [ ] Seedless Medjool or Deglet Noor dates
- [ ] Ricotta cheese
- [ ] Honey (raw and organic if possible)
- [ ] 1 ripe avocado
- [ ] 1 package ripe strawberries (frozen if out of season)
- [ ] Cacao powder (preferably raw)
- [ ] 1 can coconut milk
- [ ] Whole cane sugar (also known as Sucanat or Rapadura)
- [ ] 1 lime
- [ ] 1 lemon
- [ ] Pure maple syrup
- [ ] 8 oz sparkling water (e.g., club soda, sparkling mineral water)

best living by. This 20-percent allotment also gives you leeway when you're traveling or dining with friends, or just don't have access to the right ingredients or foods. Life requires practicality.

In the end, let this chapter mark the commencement of your journey to restore your cravings for healthier sugar. Congratulations!

Dates with Ricotta and Honey

SUGAR RESET RECIPE

The layering of sweet dates with luscious ricotta and a dollop of honey provides a wealth of texture, aromas, and flavor for your palate—a sweet and dynamite combination.

SERVES: 2–4
TOTAL TIME: 5 MINUTES

INGREDIENTS

- 2 to 3 seedless Medjool or Deglet Noor dates, split in half lengthwise
- Ricotta cheese
- Honey (raw and organic if possible)

PROCEDURE

Place a teaspoon worth of ricotta cheese in each of the date halves (or enough ricotta to fill date cavity). Drizzle with honey and enjoy!

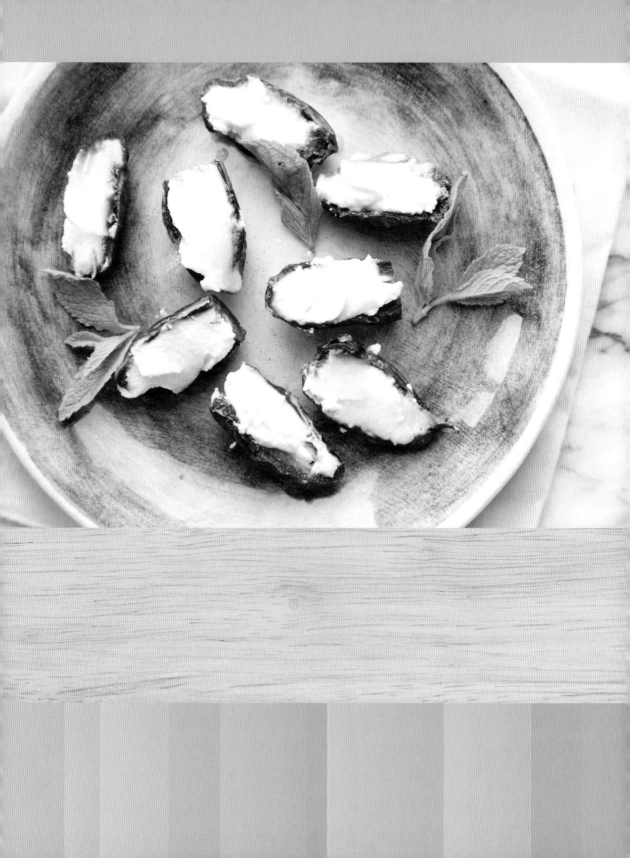

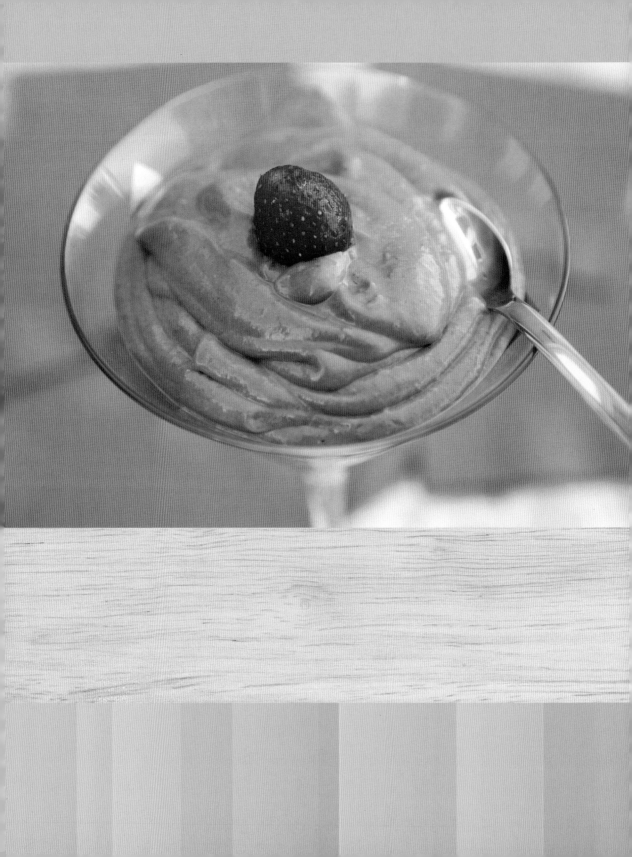

Strawberry Chocolate Mousse

This WAMP mousse recipe is so incredibly delicious you won't believe there's no refined sugar. It uses ripe strawberries and whole cane sugar to boost its sweetness.

SERVES: 2–4
TOTAL TIME: 5 MINUTES

INGREDIENTS

- 1 avocado, seed removed, quartered
- 6–7 very ripe strawberries
- 2 tbsp plus 2 teaspoons raw cacao powder
- 6 tbsp coconut milk
- 2 tbsp plus 1 teaspoon whole cane sugar
  (also known as Sucanat or Rapadura)

PROCEDURE

Place all ingredients in a blender and blend until smooth. Divide among serving bowls and enjoy!

Lemon Lime Soda

SUGAR RESET RECIPE

This homemade soda is a perfect substitute for store-bought sodas and can be made in minutes!

SERVES: 1
TOTAL TIME: 3 MINUTES

INGREDIENTS
- 2 tsp lime juice
- 2 tsp lemon juice
- 2 tsp pure Grade A maple syrup
- 8 oz sparkling water (e.g., club soda, sparkling mineral water)
- Lemon/lime rind or slices for garnish (optional)
- Ice (optional)

PROCEDURE

Add all ingredients to your favorite glass and stir to combine. Add ice if you prefer.

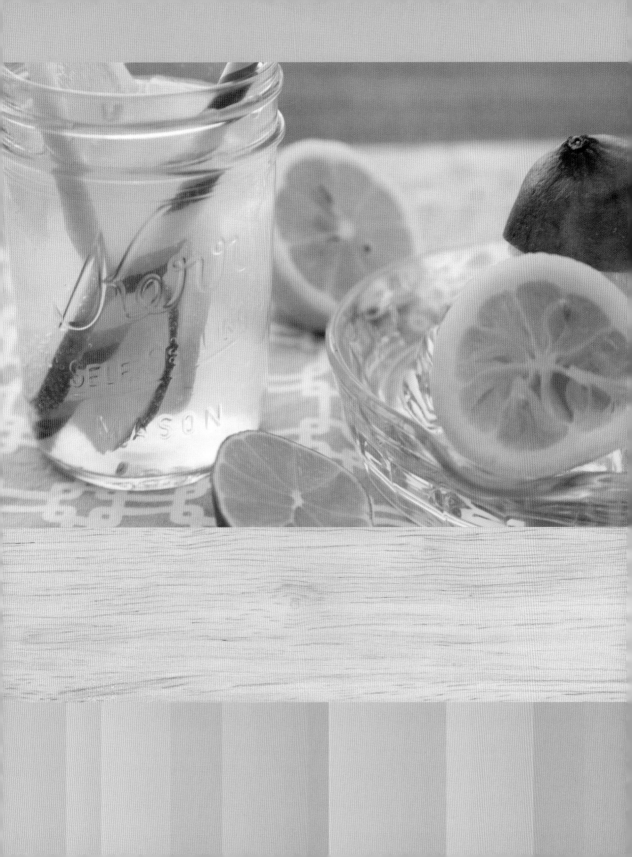

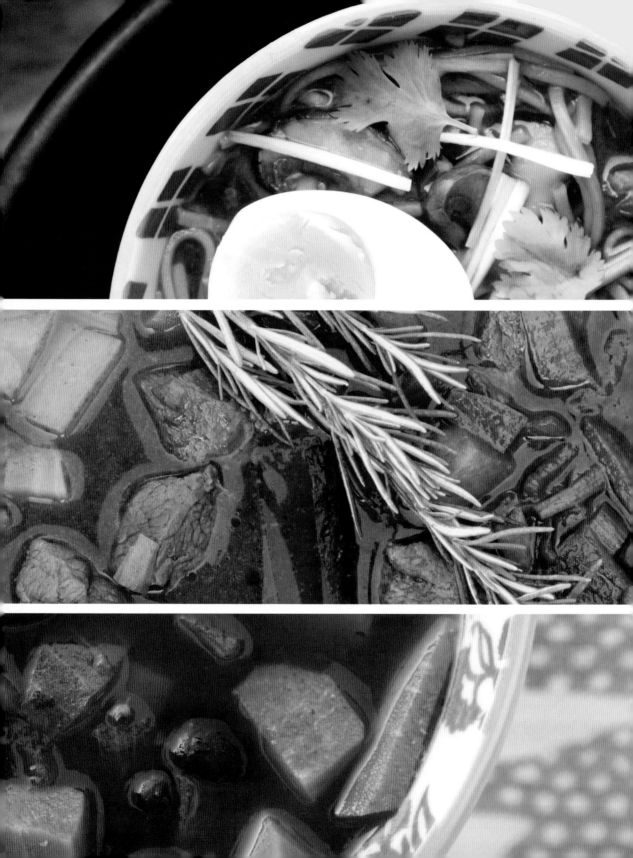

Salt
RESET

S alt, a rarefied mineral that has wielded power in war, religion, and culture for
millennia, has an illustrious history. Greek slave traders often bartered salt for
slaves, giving rise to the expression that someone was "not worth his salt." It's often said
that much of Napoleon's army died from salt deficiency and that salt helped India gain
independence from the British Empire in 1947. Nelson Mandela once famously said,
"Let there be work, bread, water, and salt for all."

Fast-forward to modern times and salt has lost its stardom. Now it's just some white
stuff in a shaker. And just as with sugar, we've lost our way when it comes to salt. The way
we eat salt today—refined and entrenched in processed foods and restaurant meals—isn't
at all the way we're meant to use it, nor is it WAMP.

Most of us are oblivious to the fact that processed salt resides in almost everything
we chew, crunch, and swallow. Food companies add salt to foods not only to make them
more appetizing, but also to mask bad flavor and influence texture. Without salt, microwave enchilada meals would taste like cardboard, or canned soup: weak and watery.

Of course, we all know that chips, pretzels, and fries are salty—the little white salt specks cling to our fingers between bites—but what about sweet foods like instant oatmeal, pancake syrup, and frosting? They're full of salt too!

Salt's even in "healthy foods" like cottage cheese and Special K. With salt in everything, it's no wonder we're eating way too much of it. Government figures suggest we're consuming almost double the amount of salt we should, our intake having increased by nearly 40 percent over the last four decades.

So, just as we did with sugar, we need to Reset our relationship with salt.

Salt of the Earth: What We Need to Know About Salt

Salt isn't the enemy. Our ancestors have been using it for ages. In early times, when humans transitioned from hunter-gatherers to agrarians, naturally salty meats began to feature less prominently in our diets. Hence, access to salt became more important. Neolithic people settled in places where they could access salt. The salt of the Dead Sea was a coveted resource, and one of the biggest reasons behind the Roman colonization of Palestine.

Salt was also one of the very first food preservatives; it was used to preserve all types of meat and fish as well as vegetables (in the form of pickling), which was especially important in times of famine, drought, or warfare. Without salt stored for these trying times, humanity may not have survived them.

Beyond basic survival, our ancestors noticed that salt made foods taste better, and they began to season foods. The Romans were very fond of using brine, a mixture of salt and water, to season their salads, which is where the name derives ("salad" comes from *sal*, Latin for "salt").

Salt was special. The Greeks thought it a divine gift. Cities near salt deposits were named in honor of it (Salzburg meaning "salt city"). The Roman army was at times paid in salt, from which the word "salary" derives (from Latin *salarium*). The Bible contains over thirty references to salt.

Incredible as it may seem, salt changed the course of history multiple times over.

But by the twentieth century, salt had evolved from special to ordinary, and from being a WAMP ingredient used sparingly in WAMP foods to a refined ingredient used

WAMP Salt

As with table sugar, the white, granulated table salt we're used to is not WAMP—it's refined, what I refer to as "processed salt." Like sugar, refined salt isn't the kind of salt our ancestors used.

The best salt to use is WAMP salt. Sea salt, for example, looks nothing like the fine, super white crystals that flow out of your salt shaker. In its true form, salt looks like crystalline rock, and can be a variety of colors from pale pink to light gray. That's because salt in its whole-food form contains a host of colorful macrominerals and trace minerals (some eighty-odd varieties). This is some good, healthy stuff. These minerals make up roughly 14 percent of WAMP salt; the remaining 82 to 86 percent consists of sodium chloride (NaCl).

The free-flowing, sandy, white salt we're using today is heavily processed—the minerals are stripped away; chemical processes are used to make it pure white; and "anticaking" agents, such as sodium aluminosilicate and magnesium carbonate, are added to ensure that it's "free flowing" (salt naturally absorbs water, so is susceptible to clumping). So this type of salt ends up containing between 97 to 99 percent sodium chloride (the rest, up to 2 percent, is usually made up of anticlumping agents and iodine), so you're just getting NaCl and none of the nutrients.

The bigger the better when it comes to WAMP salt. That's why salt mills exist, to grind less refined, rock-shaped salt. Look for the phrase "natural sea salt" or "rock salt" on labels, not "salt, calcium silicate (anticaking agent), dextrose, potassium iodide."

excessively in processed foods. The real shift began around 1950. Postwar prosperity, coupled with women increasingly finding work outside the home, spawned the need for convenience when it came to food, and two roads opened to fill it: processed foods and restaurant dining, both heavily reliant on salt, particularly processed (refined) salt.

Over the last seven decades, processed foods and restaurant eating have steadily grown, and now they make up the lion's share of our eating habits. Today, we get somewhere around 70 percent of our calories from processed foods, and nearly half the money we spend on food is spent at restaurants and other away-from-home food service outlets. Instead of using salt primarily to preserve and season WAMP dishes in our own kitchens, we've transferred the power of salting to food manufacturers and restaurant chain CEOs.

> But what about sweet foods—like instant oatmeal, pancake syrup, and frosting? They're full of salt too!

This transfer has made salt so ubiquitous in our food supply that we now end up blindly consuming way too much of it. Despite public health campaigns to raise awareness, like the FDA's "sodium education initiatives" and the "sodium" line item added to the Nutrition Facts box in 1984, we're still consuming unprecedentedly high levels of salt in our daily lives— more than 3,300 milligrams. As a comparison, scientists believe our consumption of salt in the ancient world was around 250 milligrams. The upshot of all this salt is untold risk to our bodies. According to the Harvard School of Public Health, a diet high in sodium (i.e., salt) can raise your risk of high blood pressure, heart disease, and stroke. Heart disease and stroke are the leading causes of death in the United States.

Processed Food's Best Friend

Salt is a boon to the processed-food industry. Manufacturers know that salt enhances flavor and helps to preserve food, which is key, because their products must be made, packaged, shipped, and stored before even getting to our shelves, so the longer their expiration date, the better.

But with modern research dedicated to examining this mineral, food scientists have found a whole new set of ways that salt can make factory food more appealing, and thus more sellable. Research has found that by adding salt to foods, we can enhance a slew of positive sensory attributes. For example, salt can improve the perception of a product's thickness, mask any metallic or chemical off-notes, boost the intensity of flavor, and round out overall flavor.

Salt is also used to make up for the lost flavor that results from freezing ready-made meals. It masks the bad flavors that arise from foods subjected to high temperatures or

Buyer Beware

Salt is a major determinant of thirst, and interestingly, many of the world's biggest snack companies are also the world's biggest soft-drinks companies—both epitomes of processed food. Eat their salty chips and you'll want to quench your thirst with their drinks. That's money in the bank.

long storage periods, like cereal. In beverages, particularly soft drinks, salt is used to balance the metallic aftertastes of zero- and low-calorie sweeteners or other additives. Salt is used to make sugary foods more sugary: Caramel confections and chocolate chip cookies taste sweeter when more salt is added to their formulations. This may be due to the fact that salt suppresses bitterness in food, and in doing so brings sweet flavors to the fore, or maybe due to the activation of certain sweet receptors in our mouths. Salt is also used in some meat products to "bind in water," thereby increasing product weight. That's why chickens are so big!

Salt has even spawned an entirely new class of synthetic sodium-based additives in an attempt to mimic its multifunctionality. Ingredients like sodium citrate, sodium phosphate, sodium acid pyrophosphate, disodium phosphate, sodium alginate, sodium nitrate, and sodium benzoate serve to leaven, bind, and emulsify, among other functions.

Would You Like a Side of Salt with That?

Salt's other gig is in the restaurant world: full service, fast food, and in between. Restaurant meals now account for 25 percent of our sodium intake (according to the CDC, 65 percent of sodium comes from food sold in stores). National restaurant chains are some of the worst culprits. Many entrées—at places like Olive Garden, Chili's, and Red Lobster—have levels of added salt that exceed our daily recommended limit. In order to keep us eating out, taking out, and spending our money, restaurants find it imperative to "salt to our cravings." We don't automatically think "salt" when we're biting into Domino's pepperoni pizza, P.F. Chang's egg rolls, or Chili's Honey Chipotle Ribs, yet it's loaded in all of this stuff.

Salt in Unexpected Places:
Processed Foods with Processed Salt

- Special K
- Jell-O
- Boxed cereal
- Cake mix
- Pudding
- Pancake syrup

- Frosting
- Instant oats
- Ketchup
- Raisin Bran
- Pumpernickle bread
- Canned mushrooms

- V8 Spicy Hot vegetable juice
- Canned beans
- Mozarella sticks
- Caramel
- Bran muffins

Salt opens the door to cutting corners, as it's the perfect vehicle for cheap and easy flavor. Because processed salt is relatively inexpensive and a heck of a lot more shelf-stable than herbs and spices, many times it's used in place of other, higher-quality seasonings—it replaces basil in your minestrone soup, cloves and cinnamon sticks in your lamb entrée.

Restaurants—both fast food and five-star—take even more of our power because we have no idea how much salt is being used in the kitchen. There are no labels, no stamps, no literature. We think, "OK, I'm at a nice restaurant and because there's a trained chef somewhere in the back making my food, it's *got* to have the right amount of salt." Yet, we're just going in blind and coming out blind.

Taken with a Grain of Salt: The Good News

If night after night, week after week, year after year, we rely on restaurant take-out, pizza, canned soup, and mini-bags of pretzels to feed ourselves, bad things start to happen. As with sugar, too much processed salt leads to the compromising of our taste buds. Whole, healthy, WAMP foods stop tasting good. Anything unsalted starts to taste drab, and even inedible.

The good news is that we can repair this by resetting our relationship with salt. When we start eating WAMP foods, seasoned ourselves (preferably with WAMP salt),

> ## Season to Taste
>
> It's OK to be friends with our salt shakers. The idea of "seasoning to taste" is a core concept in culinary training. There's nothing wrong with adding salt to homemade soups and stews, to season meats and other proteins, and to boost flavor in grains, for example. The key is to do it *ourselves*, with *our own two hands* and preferably with WAMP salt, so we can control the amount we put in our bodies.

our taste buds can gradually adjust. This is nothing new—in fact, in 1946, the Arctic explorer Vilhjalmur Stefansson reported that while he was living with Inuit groups who didn't add salt to their food, he first found the foods insipid and craved salt; but within a few months, he found he stopped wanting it, and when he tasted food with it, he found them unpalatable.

Eating salt the way we're supposed to can change the way we experience flavor. Fresh chicken soup starts tasting like a million bucks; summer blackberries make your mouth water. The bright, grassy flavor of parsley gets you excited. The sweetness of basil tantalizes your tongue. Your palate broadens.

When we reset ourselves to salt, most bad food—processed food—starts tasting, well, bad. Granola bars, pasta sauces, and even the canned minestrone you've always loved begin to taste egregiously salty. Even some sweet foods (which usually contain salt to boost sweetness), like chocolate chip cookies start to taste way too sweet—even harshly sweet.

Even some of your former favorite restaurant dishes will start to get on your bad side. Dishes end up tasting drastically over-seasoned. Soups and entrées get sent back (you may feel awkward and so might your waiter, but hey, it's not your fault). Believe me, it has happened to me too many times to count.

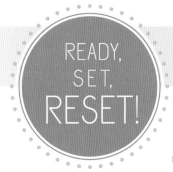

We now have a solid understanding of how we're eating the wrong kind of salt, in the wrong ways, and way too much of it.

But reading isn't enough; knowledge is only the beginning. It's time for action! The next part of this Reset asks you to eliminate foods salted by others, and instead find flavor in foods without salt, or in foods salted only by yourself, preferably with sea salt (WAMP salt).

Instructions

It works like this. For breakfast, over the next seventy-two hours, you will avoid all food with added salt, with the exception of bread (I don't exclude bread here because although it does contain salt, it's in low quantities, and bread has been baked with salt for millennia). This means you'll have to ditch cereals, breakfast wraps, and bagels. If you're not sure how much salt is in a food you'd like to eat, be a salt detective. Look at labels, check ingredient lists, and ask!

For lunch over the next three days, you'll also make a change, but this time, instead of avoiding all salted foods, you'll do your best to avoid *obviously* salty dishes: cured meats (ham, sausages) and other deli cold cuts, salad dressings, pizza, pasta dishes, soups, and sandwiches. Lunch is harder to control than our other meals, as we're usually at work or on the go. So just do your best over the next three days to minimize your intake of salty foods at lunchtime. A good rule of thumb is to avoid any foods that have over 5 percent of the daily value (DV) of sodium per serving. You can find this by looking at the Nutrition Facts box on the package.

But if you can completely avoid foods with added salt for lunch during these three days, go ahead and do so!

In between meals, you'll nix your salt consumption too. Snacks are jam-packed with high levels of sodium. Chips, crackers, trail mixes: You name it and salt's in it. Eat fresh

Don't be worried when you see "½ teaspoon" of salt in a recipe—remember, one recipe serves, on average, four people. Unless you are being advised by your medical practitioner to limit your salt intake in a certain way, these amounts are OK. For a good rule of thumb, US Dietary Guidelines recommend limiting sodium intake to less than 2,300 milligrams per day, or the equivalent of one teaspoon of salt per day.

foods like fruits, dried fruits, salads, juices, and other WAMP foods instead. Remember, dairy and meats are naturally salty foods.

For dinner, you'll be taking back control of your salt shaker and making flavorful home-cooked meals. At the end of this chapter, I've included three recipes for you to experience. Dinner is the meal in which salt intake is the highest, so I want you to tackle this head on. By cooking your own dinner using these recipes, you're not just tasting flavorful, healthy dishes based on WAMP food and empowering yourself in the kitchen; you're learning that by using your salt cellar or salt shaker, you're able to adjust salt to your tastes, and salt your food the way we're intended to: by hand, using WAMP salt, and in small quantities. You don't have to cook different recipes for each of the three days; if you like just one feel free to cook it for dinner all three days.

This salt immersion will open your eyes to how we relate to salt on a daily basis. Over the next three days, we'll get a chance to touch, taste, and discover salt all over again—a short, one-time investment that can reap huge rewards.

TIPS & TOOLS for EACH DAY

Day One

Congratulations on embarking on your first day of resetting salt! As I mentioned before, you'll want to avoid all added salt for breakfast today. Common breakfast foods that contain salt include cold cereal, cured meats (such as bacon), processed cheeses, and breakfast pastries. Bread is OK, so toast away.

Instead of eating breakfast outside the home for these first three days, you may want to cook something quick before you leave. A no-salt breakfast is easier than you think. Be creative and take this time of the day to indulge in fresh, ripe, delicious fruits, eggs, and fresh-squeezed juices. Yogurts with a fruit puree and yogurt-based smoothies are good options too.

This morning you'll notice a whole lot about salt. Your eyes will be popping out of their sockets. You'll find salt in almost all the cereal boxes in your pantry. You'll notice there's salt in the breakfast burrito you love. You'll notice added salt in places you didn't expect.

For lunch, you'll want to try your best to avoid heavily salted lunch foods such as pizza, pasta, burgers, soups, and most restaurant fare, as well as dressings and condiments that tend to contain loads of salt.

As I mentioned earlier, because we're usually eating prepared food for lunch (i.e., food from buffets or restaurants) it will be harder for you to figure out the salt content. Use your best judgment here. If you know a dish is particularly salty, like fries or hamburgers with ketchup, avoid it.

Instead, opt for dishes that are fresh and as WAMP as possible. These will naturally showcase more vegetables and fresh proteins that are bursting with flavor.

Of course, to make 100 percent sure you're avoiding loads of salt for lunch, the best course of action is to pack it from home. If you can, do so!

For dinner, you will throw on your apron and cook one of the delicious recipes from the end of this chapter. This is the fun part. These recipes are designed to impart serious flavor through the use of pungent, lively, and wonderfully fresh WAMP foods. You'll realize that with just a small amount of seasoning with sea salt on your end, WAMP meals can be extraordinary. That's because when you cook with fresh and whole foods, the flavor is unsurpassed, and by adding just a touch of salt, you get the perfect boost of flavor you're looking for instead of an overpowering salty taste.

Day Two

Today you're likely getting into the groove with breakfast. You've probably now realized how entrenched salt is in all the foods we eat—particularly every food you buy in a package or at a restaurant. You've realized that avoiding salt is extremely hard.

For lunch today, you may want to think about finding unseasoned foods like eggs, chicken, or steamed vegetables and seasoning them yourself with small amounts of salt, pepper, and butter. Soups tend to have a lot of salt, so try to avoid them as much as you can. Lunch isn't easy; just try your best here.

For dinner tonight, you might want to consider the soba-noodle dish if you haven't tried it already. It's very quick to make and introduces you to the salty flavor of Asian cuisine, in which ingredients like soy sauce, ponzu, and shoyu are used instead of white table salt. Just like salt, however, these ingredients have a lot of sodium. You'll notice in this recipe that I use only small amounts. The beauty of these ingredients is that they have a broader taste profile than straight table salt. They bring in umami, which taste experts refer to as the fifth basic taste (along with sweet, bitter, sour, and salty). Umami is a delicious, full-bodied, rich flavor that is part and parcel of Asian cuisine. It registers in the mouth as meaty and savory, similar to the flavor we get from warm, sautéed mushrooms. Bringing more umami into your kitchen automatically makes life more delicious.

Day Three

Congratulations! Only twenty-four more hours to go. On this last day, you may want to take extra time to think more about salt. Check ingredient lists of food items you may not want to eat, just for the heck of it. Take a trip to your local health food store and see what unrefined salt choices are available and restock your pantry with healthier WAMP salt.

Use today to realize that foods don't have to be seasoned with salt to taste good. In fact, realize that Mother Nature has already provided most of the flavor we need in all kinds of WAMP foods, from sweet sun-ripened fruits to fresh, sour yogurt, to spicy raw chilies, to savory sautéed mushrooms.

Fresh and dried herbs, for example, which have been used to flavor food as far back as the Iron Age, are some of nature's most divine gifts to our palates. Dill, parsley, rosemary, basil, oregano, thyme, and mint can impart a wonderful panoply of flavors, from bitter to vinegary to peppery to sweet, which can deliver more flavor power than salt ever could.

Other plant foods that deliver serious flavor are lemongrass, scallions, garlic, and shallots, as well as dried fruits and citrus zest, all highly concen-

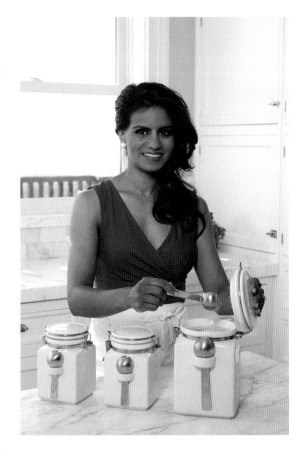

trated. Spices such as cinnamon, cloves, and cumin have been used since antiquity to add dimension and tastiness to everything from vegetables to meats to grains. Squeeze lemon in your tea and on your dishes at lunch and dinner. Add crushed fruits to your meat and other proteins. Be brave and explore!

The bottom line is that by utilizing a broader spectrum of WAMP foods, we don't need to lean on salt as much as we think we need to. Salt doesn't need to be our crutch.

Enjoy this last day of your new experience with salt.

After the Reset

After undergoing this Reset, you will most likely have experienced a serious paradigm shift in the way you think about salt.

You'll have finally opened your eyes to where salt lurks in your food—possibly for the first time ever in your life. You'll probably have realized that salt is in almost every-thing we eat—even desserts—because we're so dependent on eating out and on processed, packaged foods.

This Reset has likely empowered you in the kitchen and outside the home by forcing you to take your salting privileges back. You'll have realized that you don't need that much salt to make food taste delicious. You'll have had the chance to experience how fresh whole food can be *enhanced* by salt, not drowned out by it.

This Reset has prompted you to explore using WAMP salt in your kitchen. This type of salt is healthier, and hopefully you'll want to incorporate it into your pantry. You may also want to explore shoyu and other Asian condiments that give you a salty flavor, but with less sodium per teaspoon.

Enjoy your new relationship with salt. Your body and your taste buds will benefit for years to come.

YOUR SALT RESET GROCERY LIST

- [ ] 1 package soba noodles (8 oz or higher)
- [ ] Toasted sesame oil
- [ ] 4 oz shiitake mushrooms
- [ ] Ginger
- [ ] Mirin
- [ ] Shoyu
- [ ] Rice wine vinegar
- [ ] Scallions
- [ ] Cilantro
- [ ] 1/2 dozen eggs (optional)
- [ ] Extra-virgin olive oil
- [ ] 1 3/4 to 2 lbs lamb shoulder
- [ ] Red wine for cooking
- [ ] 2 yellow onions
- [ ] 1 garlic bulb
- [ ] Double-concentrated tomato paste
- [ ] Paprika

- [ ] Chili powder
- [ ] Ground cumin
- [ ] Cinnamon sticks
- [ ] Sea salt
- [ ] Bunch celery
- [ ] Large bunch carrots
- [ ] 1 large yellow beet
- [ ] 1 small to medium potato (optional)
- [ ] Low-sodium organic beef broth
- [ ] Fresh rosemary
- [ ] Pomegranate molasses (optional)
- [ ] Dried oregano
- [ ] Dried thyme (optional)
- [ ] Roma tomatoes (fresh or jarred/canned)
- [ ] 1 can black beans
- [ ] 1 can kidney beans
- [ ] Low-sodium organic vegetable broth

Soba Bowl

This recipe is a go-to for fast, nourishing dinners and is a perfect meal for exploring Eastern condiments such as mirin and shoyu that bring the taste of umami to foods. Although shoyu contains sodium, it is used sparingly here. You'll find this dish incomparable to restaurant soba in terms of its depth of flavor.

SERVES: 2–4
TOTAL TIME: 20 MINUTES

INGREDIENTS

- 8 oz soba noodles (100% buckwheat or buckwheat and wheat combination)
- 2 tsp toasted sesame oil
- 8 oz shiitake, crimini, or similar mushrooms, thinly sliced
- 1/2 c water
- 2 tbsp minced ginger
- 4 tbsp mirin, or to taste
- 3 tbsp plus 1 teaspoon low-sodium shoyu, or to taste
- 3 tbsp rice wine vinegar
- 3 scallions, sliced thinly on the bias
- Cilantro for garnish
- 2 hard-boiled organic eggs, sliced in half lengthwise (optional)

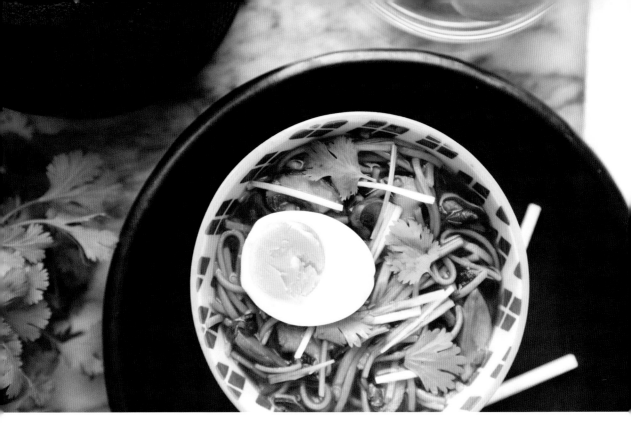

PROCEDURE

1. In a deep saucepan, bring enough cold water to cover noodles to a boil (about eight cups). Add noodles and stir immediately to prevent them from clumping together. Cook uncovered for 8 minutes or until al dente. Rinse a noodle under cold water and taste. If done, drain all noodles using a colander and rinse them under cold water. While water is running over the noodles, use your fingers to keep them separated to prevent clumping. Set aside.

2. Using the same pot, heat oil over medium heat. When hot, add mushrooms and sauté a couple of minutes, then add 1/4 cup of water, cover, and turn heat to medium-low. Cook mushrooms until fully softened—about five to eight minutes.

3. Add ginger, shoyu, rice wine vinegar, mirin, and remaining water and cook another few minutes, covered.

4. Add noodles and scallions to pot. Using tongs, toss noodles with broth.

5. Transfer noodles and broth to serving bowl. Begin to plate in individual bowls, garnish with chopped cilantro. Add half an egg to each bowl if desired.

Soba Bowl

Hearty Lamb Stew

This stew is wonderfully hearty and healthful—a wonderful example of home cooking with WAMP ingredients, using small amounts of sea salt. The rosemary and red wine provide for superb flavor.

SERVES: 8
TOTAL TIME: 50 MINUTES

INGREDIENTS

- Extra virgin olive oil
- 1 3/4 to 2 lbs lamb shoulder, fat removed, cut into large stew cubes
- 1/2 c red wine
- 1 medium sized yellow onion, small dice
- 4 garlic cloves, crushed
- 3 tbsp double concentrated tomato paste
- 1 tsp paprika
- 1 tsp chili powder
- 3/4 to 1 tsp ground cumin
- 1 cinnamon stick
- 1 tsp sea salt
- 2 stalks celery, sliced widthwise into small pieces
- 2 large carrots, peeled, cut into bite sized pieces
- 1 large yellow beat (about 10oz), peeled, cut into small cubes
- 1 small to medium sized potato, peeled, cut into small cubes (optional)
- 2 c low sodium organic beef broth
- 1–2 c water
- 1 sprig fresh rosemary
- 2 tbsp pomegranate molasses (optional)

PROCEDURE

1. Pour oil into a deep, heavy-bottomed Dutch oven or saucepan and place over high heat. When it is warm, sear the lamb pieces (a fair amount of water will be released as you go so you may not be able to sear all sides uniformly).

2. Remove lamb when done and set aside. Add wine to the pot. Let wine and remaining fat from lamb searing reduce for a few minutes, then add in onions and garlic. Lower heat to medium and cook for a few minutes.

3. Add all ingredients up to and including sea salt and continue to cook for another minute or two, stirring to combine. If ingredients are browning, add a small amount of broth.

4. Add all vegetables, water, and broth. Then add the lamb and stir to combine. If liquid does not sufficiently cover the meat, add more water. Add rosemary sprig and molasses, cover, and bring to a boil. Lower to a simmer and cook for 45 to 50 minutes or longer if you desire. When done, turn off the heat, keeping the stew covered, and let it cool for a few more minutes before serving.

Note: This stew is meant to be less thick than traditional stews. If you want more thickness, add some cornstarch, flour, or arrowroot powder. Pomegranate molasses adds a lot of flavor to this dish so if you can find it, be sure to use it!

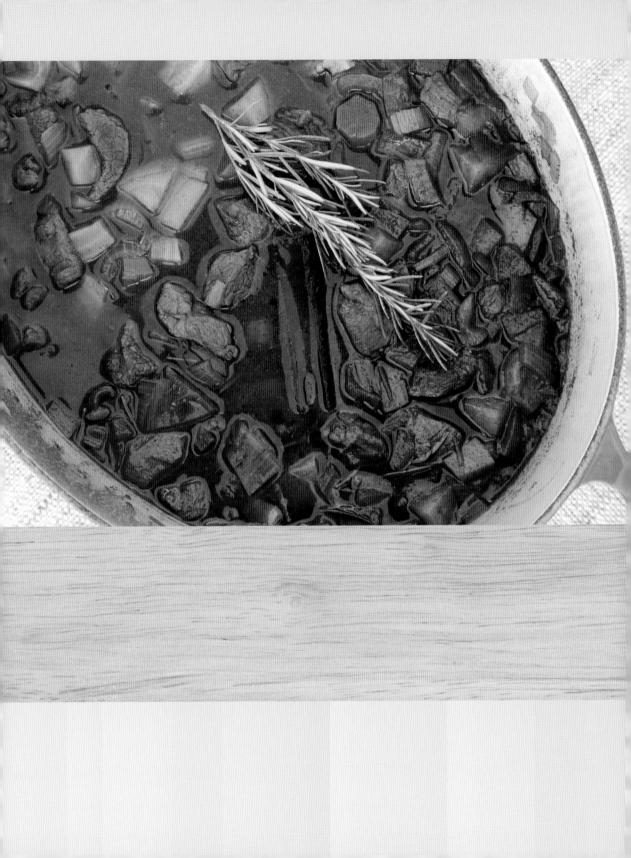

Two Bean Tuscan Soup

Prepared soups are some of the worst culprits when it comes to excessive use of processed salt. This recipe proves that its WAMP ingredients like oregano, thyme, ripe carrots and paprika—not salt—that deliver the flavors we crave.

SERVES: 4
TOTAL TIME: 20 MINUTES

INGREDIENTS

- 4 tsp extra virgin olive oil
- 10 oz red or yellow onion, small dice (about 1 large onion)
- 3 garlic cloves, finely minced
- 1 1/2 tsp sea salt
- 4 stalks celery, sliced lengthwise into 1/4 inch pieces
- 5–6 medium carrots, peeled and diced into small cubes
- 2 tbsp double concentrated tomato paste
- 1/2 tsp ground cumin
- 1 tsp paprika
- 1/2 tsp chili powder
- 1/2 tsp dried oregano
- 1/2 tsp dried thyme (optional)
- 1 c crushed, ripe roma tomatoes (fresh or jarred/canned)
- 1/2 c canned black beans
- 1/2 c canned kidney beans
- 3 c water
- 3 c low sodium organic vegetable broth

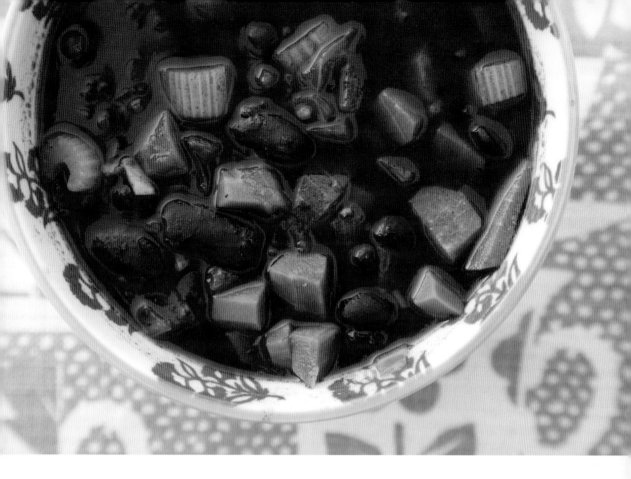

PROCEDURE

1. Place soup pot over medium-high heat. Add oil. When warm, add onions and garlic. Cook until onions begin to caramelize.

2. Add salt, vegetables, tomato paste, and spices. Cook for another few minutes. Then add crushed tomatoes and cook another couple of minutes, stirring to combine.

3. Add beans, water, and broth. Cover and bring to a boil. Lower to a simmer and cook, covered, for about 20 minutes or until carrots are sufficiently soft. Enjoy.

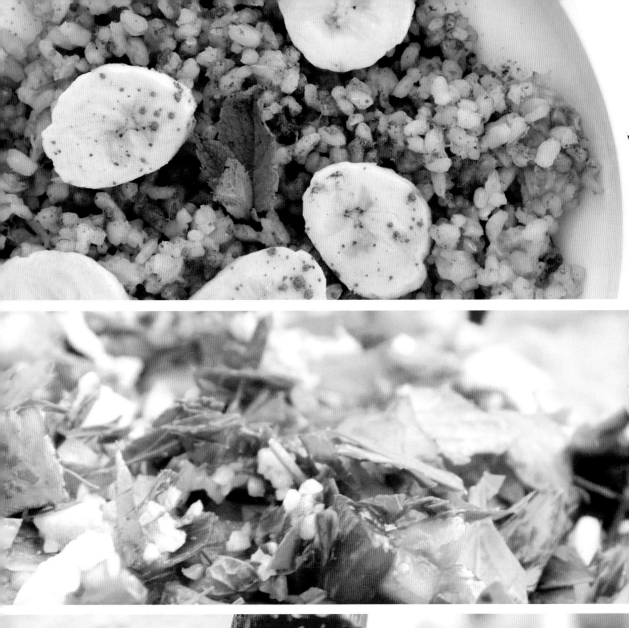
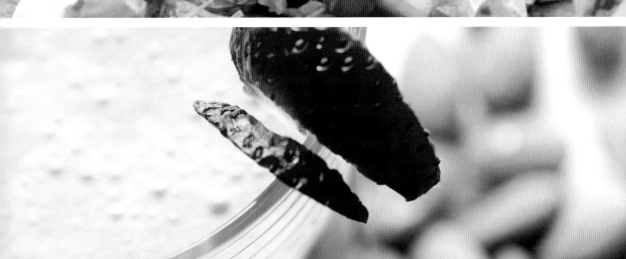

Wheat
RESET

What do rolls, crackers, wraps, burritos, bagels, pasta, cereal, toast, sandwiches, and tortillas have in common? They're all made of flour—*wheat* flour, that is. The same thing goes for French toast, baguettes, mini scones, animal crackers, wontons, vanilla wafers, dumplings, rigatoni, macaroni. . . . The list of wheat-toting foods is endless.

Have you ever thought about this? I mean, *really thought* about how this powdery white, practically tasteless ingredient can be such a big part of your everyday life? To think that it's almost impossible to avoid putting flour in your mouth at least once a day, every single day of your life, for the rest of your life, is nothing short of shocking.

Wheat is so stealthily integrated into our food that we don't realize it. No one thinks "wheat" when they're munching on fish tacos, fettuccine Alfredo, minestrone soup, or chicken parm, yet wheat flour is in all of those dishes. Wheat makes up the bulk of pizza pies, of which three billion are sold in the United States annually, but we're more focused on the bubbling cheese and toppings to notice the flat stuff holding it all together below.

Wheat flour is the main ingredient in the approximately 85 billion tortillas that are made into tacos, burritos, and enchiladas each year, but "wheat flour" is certainly not included on any menu's description—it's as if it weren't a part of the dish at all.

Without wheat flour, there would be no hot dogs, no hamburgers, no cookies 'n cream ice cream, no fortune cookies, and no Szechuan dumplings in hot sauce. Wheat has virtually penetrated every little nook, cranny, and corridor of our culinary landscape unnoticed.

Think of wheat flour as the gas for our convenience-fueled, on-the-go lifestyles. Wheat-based cereals save us countless hours in the morning; all we need to do is shake stuff into a bowl, add milk, and we're done. Who needs to cook when we have sliced bread and baguettes—the ultimate foodstuffs for grab, tear, throw-in-your-mouth eating? Wheat helps us avoid dependence on the refrigerator, stove, kitchen, and even utensils! It allows us to stash away cheap chips, crackers, and pretzels in our desk drawers, cars, and pantries for months on end.

Wheat flour practically defines not just the way we eat, but also the way we live. It's inextricable from the American lifestyle—so it's no surprise that we're eating a ton of it. In fact, we eat more wheat than any other staple food. Seventy-five percent of all grain-based products we eat in America are made of wheat, which accounts for a whopping 20 percent of all calories consumed. Corn-, rice-, and oat-based foods appear in meager proportions by comparison. And whole grains like millet, wild rice, and amaranth are consumed so little that they're not even on the USDA's radar for compiling grain statistics.

Why is this such a big deal? Wheat is *natural*, you might be thinking. It grows from the earth! What's wrong with that?

Here's what's wrong with it: This omnipresent wheat that's filling our bellies with nearly a fifth of our daily calories *isn't WAMP wheat*; it's processed wheat.

Today's wheat—and the foods it pervades—is not the same nourishing wheat of generations past, the wheat Laura and Mary helped Pa to harvest in *Little House on the Prairie*, the wheat that's the subject of so many Bible verses, the wheat that's been worshipped through the millennia by pharaohs and Roman emperors and Napoleon for its unparalleled nourishment of humanity. Rarely do we come across that kind of wheat today. Even the much-touted "whole-wheat" foods that litter grocery-store aisles these days—from whole-grain breads to cereal bars—are weak substitutes for the wheat that was eaten back in the day.

The wheat we're consuming these days is as processed and unhealthy as the white sugar packets we tackled in the Sugar Reset chapter. Wheat has been transformed into flour to serve one sole purpose: for us to eat foods that are boxed and packaged and chock-full of preservatives, flavorings, and other food-science-engineered additives.

> Seventy-five percent of all grain-based products we eat in America are made of wheat, which accounts for a whopping 20 percent of our daily calories.

So, just as with sugar, we need to take action on wheat. In order to reset ourselves back to loving healthy wheat, it's imperative we kick the processed version to the curb. That's what this very important Reset is all about.

The First Superfood: What We Need to Know About Wheat

Forget about kale; the first superfood on Earth was likely wheat. As one of the most portable, hardy, and energy-rich foods in the world, wheat has done more for the human race than any other food in history.

Around 10,000 BC, when our ancestors were transitioning from hunter-gatherers to agrarians, wheat not only helped keep them alive, it helped them thrive. With the newfound understanding of how to intensively farm plants, food availability came more solidly under human control. From a population of less than 10 million, the human race exploded, a lot of it because of calories from wheat.

Wheat has been revered by some of the most iconic thinkers in history. One of the first texts to tout the importance of wheat was the Code of Hammurabi in Babylon, where it was so important it required taxation. The Bible counts wheat as one of the "Seven Species" of the Land of Israel, along with barley, grapes, wine, olives, figs, and pomegranates. Wheat was thought to be so vital to life that the Greeks offered it to the goddess Demeter. The Romans called her Ceres, a name from which the word "cereal" derives. Wheat was even mentioned in Plato's *Republic* (380 BC): "And for their nourishment [men] will provide meal from their barley and flour from their wheat, and roasting and kneading these they will serve noble cakes and loaves on some arrangement of reeds or clean leaves."

Its concentrated source of nourishment for armies made wheat a critical weapon in times of war. According to Socrates, "No man qualifies as a statesman who is entirely ignorant on the problems of wheat." Even the Civil War was considered a victory of bread (i.e., wheat) over cotton.

Wheat was once our superhero—the Batman of food. But that's changed, and we're no longer rolling out the red carpet to worship it, in large part because it's not the same stuff. It's not WAMP.

The Wheat Berry

Given that we rarely, if ever, eat wheat in its natural, untouched form, it's probably helpful to make sure we have a solid understanding of what it really is. What are those "amber waves of grain"? Funny enough, real wheat looks nothing like a loaf of bread, a bag of flour, or the stuff you pour into a cereal bowl.

Wheat, in its most basic state, looks like a smooth, nutty-brown-colored puffed piece of grain. This kernel, also known as the wheat berry, can be found at the tip of those long, billowy, yellow-golden blades of grass you midwesterners may have seen whizzing past you as you were doing eighty-five miles per hour on the highway. (Yeah, you know what I'm talking about.)

Humankind first stumbled upon wheat around the dawn of the Neolithic era somewhere near the Karacadag Mountains in southeastern Turkey. This ancient kind of wheat was likely called einkorn wheat, a grass that contains the identical genetic fingerprint of modern domesticated wheat. Our ancestors probably examined the stalk, and upon discovering a raw kernel at the tip, did nothing more than pop it into their mouths and chewed: tough and probably not so yummy, but definitely a food to be explored.

As people found better ways—likely through trial and error—to separate the grain from the ears, and crush and crack the whole kernel by hand using millstones and stone querns to produce the first forms of wheat flour, one of the very first minimally processed ingredients in human history, wheat started to unveil its glorious potential as a perfect ingredient for simple, nourishing dishes. People soon realized that adding a bit of water to wheat flour made a porridge that delivered not only sustained energy but a good deal of hearty protein too.

It was likely in this way that we were consuming wheat until about 4000 BC when, either through yeast spores accidentally finding their way into dough, or possibly when ale instead of water was used to mix the dough, the ancient Egyptians accidentally discovered how to make bread that rose upon baking. Leavened bread had officially arrived, and with it, wheat would become a priceless, saint-like ingredient. Grinding grains would become part of a household's daily routine, and porridge, bread, and even wheat noodles (which may have been an invention of the ancient Chinese around 1700 BC) would define wheat foods—all of them perfectly WAMP.

What a Grind: The Romans Take Over

It wouldn't be until the time of the ancient Athenians and Virgil's *Aeneid* that wheat would become just a tad adulterated. The invention of rotary stone mills (rotary querns) and later water mills (circa 85 BC) made grinding wheat kernels the job of animals instead of human hands but more significantly, helped remove the outer layer of the kernel, called the bran. The Romans loved the idea and took the separation further by inventing sieves out of horsehair or papyrus, which they found could better sift out more of the tough bran and help make the flour softer and much lighter. The only difference was that a bit of nourishment was lost—the bran harbored lots of fiber and vitamins.

For the next two thousand years, as grinding and sifting innovations continued, wheat flour got even finer, allowing even greater removal of the bran. Millers went so far as to regrind the flour, passing the wheat through mills multiple times to further break down the kernel into finer and finer grinds. At this point, the bran could almost be completely removed from the kernel. But nothing else had changed. Wheat was, for all intents and purposes, still a WAMP food.

Wheat's Fall from Grace

"If it ain't broke, don't fix it" is how the saying goes. But unfortunately, that wasn't the fate for wheat.

Refined Wheat vs. WAMP Wheat

A "refined" grain refers to grain that has been altered in ways that change it from its natural state, which generally involves the removal of the bran and germ, leaving only the endosperm. These three components make up a whole wheat berry. With two important pieces missing, a majority of the grain's original nutrients are lost. (In this book, I refer to refined wheat as processed wheat.)

According to some studies, as much as 75 percent of phytochemicals are lost when wheat is refined. Studies now reveal that eating whole-grain wheat flour (WAMP wheat!) vs. refined wheat flour can lower the risk of countless chronic diseases, including stroke, type 2 diabetes, heart disease, and colorectal cancer, while supporting weight maintenance and healthy blood pressure levels.

Wheat's fall from grace started with the invention of the roller mill around 1870—a feat of engineering that resulted in refined, or processed, wheat for the first time. With this new technology, stone grinding was replaced by industrial steel (and sometimes iron or porcelain) grinding, which not only provided a finer flour and cleaner separation of the bran from the kernel but also removed the germ for the first time in history—the most nutritious part of the wheat berry. Since the germ tended to taint the color of flour (making it yellowish gray because of its carotene content) and contained oils that caused flour to oxidize and go rancid about as quickly as milk went sour, people thought this new and completely refined wheat flour was flat-out genius. Now, with its lengthened expiration date, wheat flour could be shipped from a factory afar instead of milled locally, was beautifully bright white, and could last for months.

But with all these bells and whistles came a price. Wheat flour lost all of its healthy goodness. With the bran and germ now completely eradicated, wheat flour was no longer a WAMP food. B vitamins, protein, fiber, and countless other nutrients (vitamins, iron, magnesium, copper, unsaturated fat, etc.) were all gone.

As we progressed through the twentieth century, wheat became even more processed,

> Over the last one hundred years, foods made of wheat have gone from being nutritional powerhouses, made simply and by hand, to factory products as processed and nutritionally empty as a Twinkie.

and alarm bells started to go off. Studies found that refined flour was likely the cause of the deficiency-related diseases beriberi (vitamin B1 deficiency) and pellagra (niacin deficiency), so the U.S. government mandated that flour and breads be enriched with nutrients. But of course, as we know from the chapter on The Power of WAMP, that's never as nourishing as the real thing. And as bigger and better industrialized mills and more technology were developed, the conversion of wheat berries to flour became a complex, high-tech process.

These days, kernels are subjected to extremely high temperatures (thanks to the high speed of the steel roller mills) and separated and tempered—all in an effort to obtain flour with the perfect crumb, texture, shape, color, shelf life, and flavor. We have even gone so far as to bleach flour with chemicals to make it lighter, and at one point added potassium bromate to improve its "spring" (although today the trend has reversed, with most flour products claiming they're "unbleached" and "unbromated").

Sadly, less than 2 percent of the wheat flour we now consume per year is truly WAMP. The rest is all refined. If you were to plop down a five-pound bag of white "all-purpose" in front of an Egyptian, Israelite, or Athenian of the ancient world, they wouldn't have a clue what they were looking at.

Processed Food Depends on Processed Wheat

As with sugar and salt, wheat flour is the perfect base for unhealthy food. If we add salt, sugar, fat, some preservatives, and flavoring to refined flour, we get a myriad of processed

How Wheat Is Converted to Flour

Ancient, WAMP Wheat Flour

- Crush and grind wheat kernels into flour using millstones, rotary mills, or windmills.

Modern, Processed Wheat Flour

- Wheat goes through a cleaning process at the "cleaning house."

- Passes through magnetic separator.

- Passes through a separator.

- Passes through an aspirator.

- Passes through a destoner.

- Passes through a disc-separator.

- The wheat is "tempered": Moisture is added in precise amounts to toughen the bran and mellow the inner endosperm.

- Grinding process begins: The modern milling process is a gradual reduction of the wheat kernels through grinding and sifting. Kernels are fed from bins to roller mills, corrugated cylinders made from chilled steel. The paired rolls rotate inward against each other, moving at different speeds. Passing through the corrugated "first break," rolls begin the separation of bran, endosperm (starch), and germ.

- Sifting process: Inside the sifter, there may be as many as twenty-seven frames, each covered with either a nylon or stainless-steel screen, with square openings that get smaller and smaller the farther down they go.

- Bleaching: Flour is exposed to chlorine gas or benzoyl peroxide to whiten and brighten color.

- Wheat is enriched: Iron and B vitamins riboflavin, niacin, and thiamine are added as well as malt for flavor and to increase loaf height.

foods to munch on. This is the stuff that floods the middle section of your local grocery store (and your own middle). Processed wheat has spawned an entirely new array of food that would make Homer himself roll over in his grave. Walk down the snack aisle, cereal aisle, or practically any aisle at the supermarket and you'll likely find "wheat flour" on the ingredient list of hundreds of items, from breakfast bars to crackers. Because processed wheat flour is such an inexpensive and versatile food input, it has become the perfect match to the processed-food industry's needs; it makes everything from Pop-Tarts to Girl Scout cookies possible.

> People thought this new and completely refined wheat flour was flat-out genius. But with the bran and germ now completely eradicated, B vitamins, protein, fiber, and countless other nutrients were all gone.

Good Luck Finding a Truly Whole-Wheat, WAMP Product

I love whole wheat, but it's incredibly hard to find, even in the biggest of cities. Over the course of the last several years, there's been a resurgence in the need to get back to wheat's roots and provide whole-grain-wheat foods to the American public. There's no doubt that these foods are healthier, but there's a hitch: True WAMP wheat foods are a rarity. That's because, ironically, whole-wheat flour shares the same problem as refined wheat flour: It's found mainly in processed foods. When you see "whole wheat" on an ingredient list, it will in most instances be accompanied by words like "corn syrup," "soybean oil," "fructose," and "dextrose." Next time you visit your grocery store, take a look at where "whole wheat" turns up. You'll notice that the majority of the time it's in muffins, buns, energy bars, cereal bars, pancake mix, crackers, cereals, and other prepared and packaged foods that are *also* full of sugars, salts, and fats.

Strangely enough, according to the Whole Grain Council, the fastest-growing segments of whole-grain food items in stores today are snack foods and patisserie—that's stuff like scones, cakes, and cookies. How are these wholesome? A frosted, sugary scone is a frosted sugary scone, regardless of whether it's made with whole-wheat flour or not.

WAMP Bread Is Hard to Find

When refined flour is made into an ancient food like bread, bad things happen. Modern bread isn't the same as ancient bread. No longer are most breads made with just four simple, wholesome ingredients (whole-wheat flour, water, yeast, and salt). Now sugar, dough conditioners, vinegar, and oil, as well as a whole array of food-processing inputs, have joined the party. Bread has been corrupted.

Finding *true* whole-wheat bread isn't easy. The next time you're in a store, see what you can find. You'll notice that whole-wheat breads aren't made with *just* whole wheat. Instead, whole-wheat flour is usually married to refined flour, which means your bread isn't a WAMP food after all.

When choosing wheat bread, look for those four ingredients listed above: whole wheat, salt, yeast, and water. If you see these in the bread you're interested in, you can be assured you're eating a WAMP wheat product: 100 percent whole-wheat bread.

Best of all, this kind of bread is guaranteed to make your taste buds sing. It's nuttier, richer, and much more flavorful. It's how we were meant to enjoy wheat!

Ancient WAMP Bread Ingredients
Fresh stone-ground whole-wheat flour, water, sourdough starter (i.e., yeast), salt

Modern Processed Bread Ingredients
Enriched Flour (Wheat Flour, Barley Malted Flour, Niacin, Iron-Reduced, Thiamine Mononitrate [Vitamin B1], Riboflavin [Vitamin B2], Folic Acid [Vitamin B]), Water, High-Fructose Corn Syrup, Yeast, Salted Butter. Contains 2 percent or less of the following: Salt, Wheat Gluten, Whey, Beta-Carotene, Flavor(s) Natural Butter, Vinegar, Soybean(s) and/or Cottonseed Oil, Honey, Soy Lecithin, Yeast Nutrients (Monocalcium Phosphate, Calcium Sulphate [Sulfate], Ammonium Sulfate), Corn Starch, Dough Conditioner(s) (Contains one or more of the following: Sodium Stearoyl Lactylate, Mono- and Diglycerides), Guar Gum, Calcium Propionate (Preservative).

Nabisco Honey Maid Graham Crackers

Unbleached enriched flour (**wheat flour**, niacin, reduced iron, thiamine mononitrate [vitamin B1], riboflavin [vitamin B2], folic acid), graham flour (**whole-grain wheat flour**), sugar, soybean oil, honey, calcium carbonate (source of calcium), salt, baking soda, maltodextrin, cinnamon, soy lecithin. Contains: wheat, soy.

A quest for whole-wheat cereal is equally taxing. Even in the cases where you might find "whole-wheat grain" (i.e., not flour but the wheat kernel) on an ingredient list—which happens most in the cereal aisle—you'll be surprised to know that this could mean serious processing too. Some of the most popular cereals on the market, such as Shredded Wheat and Grape Nuts, use serious feats of engineering, including gun puffing and extrusion (where whole-wheat kernels are subjected to extremely harsh heat and pressure and forced through tiny holes to form shapes like letters, O's, and clovers—all of which strip the nutrition right out).

Meanwhile, in our effort to obtain versatile, hardy, abundant, and cheap wheat to fuel our desire for bagels by the boatload, pancakes by the stack, and pizzas by the billions, agricultural scientists have tinkered with the genetic code of wheat so much that the kind of grass that's being harvested today is very different from the genetic code of original wheat. With all the crossbreeding and hybridization, wheat has evolved into a plant that has a lot more gluten (the proteins that allow for perfectly plumped bagels and chewy dough) and a lot less nutrition than it would if it were allowed to evolve naturally.

So, not only are we contending with refined wheat and wheat in processed foods, we're also dealing with wheat that may be neither safe nor aptly suited for our bodies.

Expanding Your WAMP Grain Horizons

Eating WAMP wheat isn't easy. We've just learned all about that. So, why don't we expand our horizons and instead start paying attention to wheat's whole grain brethren: rice, quinoa, and the entire cast of whole-grain characters? At the same time our

> According to U.S. government statistics, at the turn of the twentieth century, home baking accounted for 90 percent of flour consumption. This means we were making most wheat-based foods at home. By 1990, however, less than 10 percent of wheat flour consumption occurred at home, a tip-off to the fact that we had started eating wheat almost exclusively in the form of processed food.

Neolithic ancestors found wheat, they also came across barley. And after that, millet, spelt, rice, and corn. If you look around the globe today, these types of whole grains, collectively with wheat, provide the largest amount of food energy to our species. Instead of eating 75 percent of grains in the form of wheat, why not spread the love?

Barley is as old as wheat—one of the three Neolithic founder crops grown in the Fertile Crescent—and has a wondrous flavor when seasoned and prepared in soups and stews. Millet, a butter-hued, tiny whole grain, has been used throughout Asia and Africa for hundreds of years. It's made into delectable flat breads and porridges that are sweetened with cream, milk, and honey as well as vegetables.

Farro is one of my all-time favorite WAMP grains. It's a beautifully bronze-hued grain that resembles rice, and when cooked, puffs up into gorgeously nutty, chewy, and warming bits of delight that, when paired with bananas and cinnamon, will make your mouth sing.

Cornmeal, known as polenta in Italy or grits in the South, is another WAMP grain we should take the time to admire. It's just a whole corn kernel, dried and ground down. With its beautiful, bright yellow hue and unique texture it's a mouthwatering base for

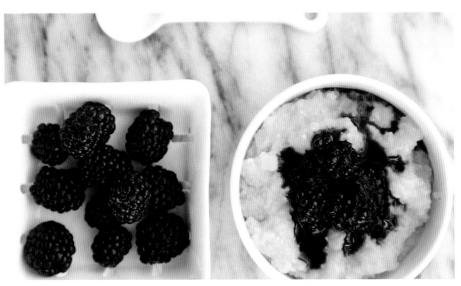

Cooked cornmeal is a WAMP grain that pairs well with sweet fruits and sauces

many sweet cereals, porridges, and side dishes. The Italians fry polenta into crispy, golden fritters, layer it with fresh goat and sheep cheeses with fresh spicy tomato-basil sauces, and nestle it into braised proteins.

Quinoa (pronounced KEEN-wah), although technically not a cereal, is considered a whole grain too—it's a powerful, nutrient-packed food first cultivated by the Incas, who referred to it as their "mother grain." Quinoa is a naturally gluten-free grain and unlike wheat it is considered one of a very few plant-based "complete" proteins. Quinoa was to the Incas what wheat is to us Americans. It comes in red, black, and golden-yellow color and cooks faster than almost all grains—in about twelve to fifteen minutes. Eating quinoa, especially when paired with avocados and salsa, is extraordinary. It's filling yet fluffy and light, crunchy yet soft, a little like couscous but with a more sophisticated and nuttier flavor profile.

WAMP grains, when paired with fresh ingredients and seasonings, are marvelous, delectable little creatures. To rob ourselves of this pleasure and focus only on wheat would be a huge loss.

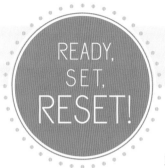

Let's repair this dysfunctional relationship with wheat once and for all. The only way to do this is by living it: putting everything we've learned into practice and putting our taste buds to work. Reading isn't enough; in order to successfully restore our love for healthy wheat, we must see, touch, and taste.

As with the Sugar and Salt Resets, this Reset is based not only on discovering new flavors but also on deleting the wrong foods from our lives. The deleting aspect is extremely important, because it forces us to become more aware of the way we're eating. Keep this in mind as you head into this important Reset.

Instructions

Here's what you'll do. For three consecutive days, you'll avoid wheat *in all forms*, with the exception of the recipes listed below. This means most breads, pastas, cereals, crackers, and sandwiches will be off limits. This will require that you examine ingredient lists on packages or ask wait staff and others who prepare your food what's in it. Be vigilant! Know what you're eating and give it your all.

To help you fend off wheat, see the Wheat Cheat Sheet to the right. Be careful because there are also many foods you may not think contain wheat, but do.

Read packages carefully, and if you see the word "wheat" anywhere, that food's off-limits. This includes all whole-wheat foods, because, as discussed above, finding 100 percent whole-wheat foods is no easy task.

If you are feeling challenged, remember: This isn't about giving up pizza, bread, and lasagna for the rest of your life; it's about becoming *aware* over the course of three days. By investigating, thinking, handling, and asking, this Reset will make a lightbulb go off in your head. You'll have many "oh, wow" moments as you go through these three days.

In exchange for shaking off processed wheat, you'll fill your belly with some

Spotting Wheat: Your Cheat Sheet

- All baked goods: pastry, muffin, cookies, brownies, cakes, cupcakes, etc.
- Bran
- Couscous
- Crepes
- Croutons
- Durum
- Einkorn
- Emmer
- Enriched flour
- Farro
- Flour
- Gnocchi
- Hard Red Spring
- Muffins
- Seitan
- Semolina
- Soba (100 percent buckwheat is okay)
- Stone-ground wheat
- Tortillas: tacos, burritos, enchiladas
- Udon
- Unbleached flour
- Unbromated flour
- Wheat breads: sourdough, ciabatta, baguette, whole-grain wheat, multigrain, seven-grain, raisin bread, etc.
- Wheat germ
- All types of wheat pasta
- Whole Wheat
- Wraps

fantastic WAMP grains instead. I've included four simple recipes that will activate your taste buds and bring a smile to your face. Because wheat is hidden in nearly every meal and morsel of our day, I've provided recipes to nourish you for breakfast, lunch, and dinner. Try the Banana-Cinnamon Rice Cereal in the morning. It's quick to cook, energizing, and really filling, so it's great fuel for those who routinely need a big bowl of cereal for breakfast. You may want to try the tabouli recipe on its own as a salad or along with a protein of your choice for lunch—it's a great alternative to sandwiches.

Wheat Wording

The word "wheat" is found on food labels in many forms. It's important to know what means WAMP and what doesn't. Here's a cheat sheet:

- "Whole wheat bread": This doesn't necessarily mean the bread is made solely of whole wheat; it could also have refined/processed wheat. Investigate the ingredient list further. (See sidebar on page 100.)

- "100% whole wheat bread": A WAMP wheat product.

- "Wheat flour (unbromated, unbleached)": This is not WAMP wheat. It means the product is made of refined wheat flour. The word "whole" is not used.

- "Whole grain wheat flour" or "whole wheat flour": WAMP wheat is used. But make sure there aren't other processed and refined ingredients in the ingredient list.

- "Enriched wheat flour": Processed wheat enriched with isolated nutrients. This product is not WAMP.

The quinoa dish is a guaranteed crowd-pleaser. It's hearty but light at the same time and with the avocado dressing it provides fresh, healthy fat, and is perfect as a protein-packed vegetarian meal.

You may find that you can easily eschew wheat over these three days without needing my recipes as substitutes, but I highly recommend using them anyway. It's the only way you will discover the amazing flavor in WAMP wheat and other whole-grain wheat alternatives. Remember, eating healthy is all about *loving* to eat healthy!

TIPS & TOOLS for EACH DAY

Ditching wheat can change your life. Here are some day-by-day tips for making the most of this essential Reset.

Day One

Good morning! Congratulations on embarking on the first day of this very important Reset. Because processed wheat loves breakfast, you will get activated from the get-go. Take a look at your cereal box. Is "wheat" on the ingredient list? No toast or bagels this morning, no pancakes or waffles.

If you religiously stop at the coffee shop on your way to work, obviously all breakfast pastries and treats are off-limits—croissants, scones, muffins, and doughnuts. Breakfast burritos are wheat-based too.

If you have some time in the morning, get to your kitchen and prepare the banana cereal recipe or something else that you're used to making such as scrambled eggs or a quick omelet. Sautéed spinach with mushrooms is quick and lovely in the morning, especially with sundried tomatoes. If you're short on time, try a smoothie or some fruit. If you love to get up with a warm bowl of oatmeal, you don't need to change a thing!

Lunch will be a big eye-opener for many of you, as you'll quickly realize how wheat makes our food convenient, cheap, portable, and even utensil-free. Lunchtime go-to's like sandwiches, pizza, stuffed pitas, hamburgers, hot dogs, subs, and burritos can all be eaten with nothing more than your own two hands (and maybe napkins if you like to keep it clean).

So you'll find that things can get a bit sticky, but no need to worry. You have a lot of room to maneuver. Wraps and sandwiches will have to wait, but you can enjoy what's in between the buns and tortillas. You can load up on salads (without the croutons, of course), and meats here to help make up for any fuel you may lose from bread, noodles, or pastas.

What you'll quickly realize is that you won't be able to eat much without a fork, knife, or spoon, which can be a good thing. Choose freshly made WAMP foods like bean and rice dishes, lots of vegetable dishes, and animal proteins (go for pasture-raised poultry and meat when you can, they're SUPER WAMP foods). For lunch, basically think fresh fruits, vegetables, rice, and protein. Another tip: Try sticking to Asian cuisines that focus on rice instead of wheat—Japanese, Korean, Vietnamese, Indian.

Snack attacks will also keep you on your toes today. Wheat Thins, Ritz Crackers, breadsticks, pretzels, and graham crackers are all wheat bombs. This is your time to make the changes you've wanted to make! Instead of munching on these pitfalls to get energy, try a fresh-squeezed juice or coconut water to keep you going, or a hot cup of loose-leaf green or black tea with lemon and honey. Plain yogurt with some honey, or a boiled egg are both good high-protein options. In most instances, snacking may not even be due to hunger. Try taking a walk or even meditating for a few minutes.

So, what's for dinner today? This meal may end up being the easiest for a lot of you, as it's usually protein heavy. This may be a good time to try some paleo recipes you've wanted to explore, or gluten-free recipes. Today might be a good day to cook the quinoa portion of the recipe below (sans the avocado dressing), as it keeps well for several days and will save you time, or perhaps cook a pot of brown rice for the Banana-Cinnamon Rice Cereal tomorrow. Tonight might be a good night to also cook the Tabouli recipe for tomorrow's lunch—it's quick and easy and stores well.

Day Two

Day two will be much easier since you've now scoped out the scene. Breakfast will probably be a lot easier than yesterday. You've likely realized how much processed wheat dominates this first meal of the day. Try getting creative with it in order to fight back. Yogurt with some crushed fruit or last night's leftovers are good ideas. Of course, you can have the cereal again, too! Feel free to check out the Breakfast Reset for more recipe ideas. Breakfast should be fresher, brighter, and more flavorful than the usual toast and jam or cereal with milk.

If you found a wheat-free lunch yesterday that worked for you, stick to it. Otherwise, you might want to set aside some time this morning to pack your lunch. Using proteins left over from the day before (chicken, boiled eggs, steak), mixed with some fresh greens, chopped carrots, radishes, avocado, and parsley or cilantro, is an easy dish to pack for work. Just add a simple dressing on top, and you're good to go.

> Brown rice is one of the best and easiest whole grains to substitute for processed wheat. If you don't own a rice cooker, pop two cups of brown rice into a saucepan along with four cups of water, and cook, covered, for about forty minutes. You'll have enough rice to last you the next several days. Now may also be a good time to try to invest in a rice cooker, which makes cooking rice comically simple. I love the Zojirushi brand.

Be on the lookout today for wheat snacks and processed foods that lurk in your usual surroundings. Take a few minutes to check your office pantry or your pantry at home. Sun Chips, cereal bars, Goldfish crackers, and practically everything that makes crumbs after the first bite is wheat-based.

For dinner tonight, you may want to try making the quinoa recipe below. It is very quick and extremely filling, perfect for a family. Soba noodles are also a good idea for dinner if you're craving pasta. Just try to find the 100 percent buckwheat version if you can. Asian cuisine is still a good take-out choice. Just remember to skip the roti or naan with your Indian entrées.

You've also probably noticed by now how difficult it is to find desserts that aren't made of wheat. Cookies, cakes, biscotti, pie, muffins, scones—you name it—are all made of processed wheat.

Instead, try eating a small piece of a dark chocolate bar (70 percent or higher cacao content). It's a beautiful way to satisfy a sweet tooth in a small package! You can also try ripe peaches or pears drizzled with honey or maple syrup.

Day Three

Hey, look at you! You made it through the last forty-eight hours! You only have one more day to go, and you're going to breeze through it.

Today, take a few minutes at mealtimes to note the epiphanies you've already had—they will astound you.

Breakfast will be a breeze by now. If you've left the cereal recipe until today, this will be an exciting dish to experience. If you've left the tabouli recipe until today, too, make sure you get to it. It's a cherished mezze (or small plate) dish throughout the Middle East and usually served alongside hummus and baba ganoush. Tabouli consists of bulgur wheat, which is made by cracking and parboiling whole-wheat kernels (in this process, usually only a small amount of the bran is removed). So bulgur is minimally altered, hence a WAMP wheat.

> Don't think of it as a sacrifice as much as an opportunity to listen to your body and discover patterns and habits in your eating that you weren't aware of before.

You'll probably have realized by now too that French and Italian cuisines are off-limits during this Reset period. Minestrone soup, bread, calzones, baguettes, gnocchi, pizza—they're all made of refined wheat flour. Take this period of eschewing French and Italian to explore cuisines you haven't in the past. The flavors of ethnic cuisine work wonders to awaken our taste buds and senses.

This is the last day the bakery will be off-limits to you. But don't think of it as a sacrifice as much as an opportunity to listen to your body, your habits, and your rhythms. These three days are the ideal time to start getting in tune with your body and discovering patterns and habits in your eating that you weren't aware of before.

Finish off the day strong and be extra proud of yourself for what you've done to reset your relationship with wheat!

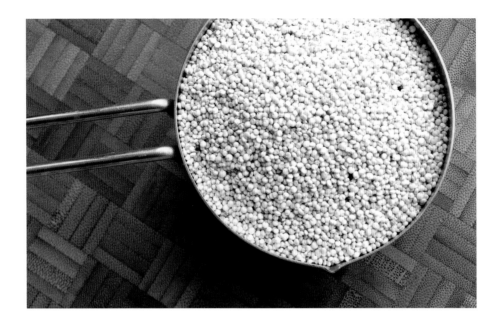

After the Reset

You did it! No processed wheat for seventy-two hours, plus an introduction to WAMP whole-grain recipes. You've accomplished a lot in a little time. After this Reset, you've likely changed the way you will eat wheat *for the rest of your life*.

By diving in headfirst and eliminating processed wheat for three days, you've learned just how much our culture depends on this nutrient-depleted food and how it shows up in every meal of the day. You know now that snacking on packaged foods is synonymous with consuming processed wheat.

Meanwhile, these three days have clued you into some amazing WAMP cuisine! These new dishes, flavors, and textures will propel you toward delicious whole grains that heretofore you may have ignored.

You are now truly ready to make serious changes to how you eat wheat. You may decide to switch up breakfast, or you may change the way you select snacks at the grocery store, or how you order lunch at your favorite restaurant.

Embrace these changes, give yourself a pat on the back, and keep exploring!

YOUR WHEAT RESET GROCERY LIST

- [ ] Pasture butter (or organic butter)
- [ ] 1 banana
- [ ] 1 c brown rice
- [ ] Ground cinnamon
- [ ] Unsweetened almond milk or organic/grass-fed cow's milk (optional)
- [ ] 1 c quinoa
- [ ] Organic expeller-pressed canola oil, olive oil, or coconut oil
- [ ] Ground cumin
- [ ] Ground coriander
- [ ] Chili powder
- [ ] Sea salt
- [ ] 1 can organic pinto beans
- [ ] 1 red bell pepper

- [ ] 2 ripe organic avocados
- [ ] 2 limes
- [ ] 1 serrano chili
- [ ] 1 package coconut palm sugar or unrefined cane sugar (see page 61 for list)
- [ ] #1 bulgur (or "fine bulgur")
- [ ] 1 bunch scallions
- [ ] 1 small yellow onion
- [ ] 2 small, ripe tomatoes
- [ ] 2 bunches fresh mint
- [ ] 2 bunches flat-leaf parsley
- [ ] 2 lemons
- [ ] Ground pepper
- [ ] 1 bunch small, crisp romaine lettuce

Banana-Cinnamon Rice Cereal

Cinnamon and banana is a winning combination, but when warmed and mixed with the nutty goodness of whole grain brown rice, it's to die for. This recipe is here as the perfect substitute for boxed cereal. If the rice is made ahead of time, this recipe can be made in minutes. If you'd like to cut your time down even further, you may skip the butter and simply heat all ingredients in a bowl in the microwave.

SERVES: 1–2
TOTAL TIME: 10 MINUTES

INGREDIENTS

- Pasture butter to coat pan
- 1 ripe banana, sliced into 1/4 inch thick discs
- 1 c cooked brown rice
- 1/2 tsp ground cinnamon (extra to taste)
- Unsweetened almond milk or cows milk, pasture-raised if possible (optional)

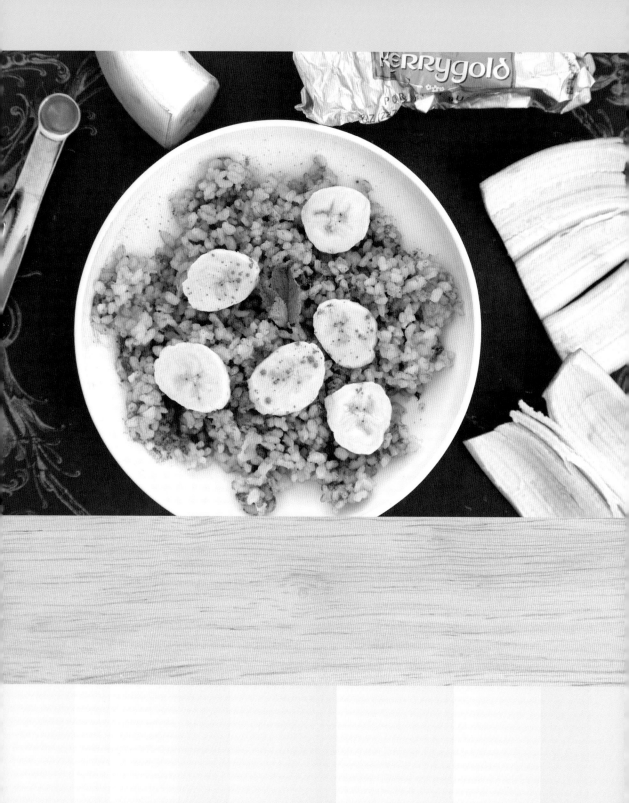

PROCEDURE

1. Heat the frying pan over low to medium heat and lightly coat the surface with a small amount of butter.

2. Add banana slices, spreading them across the surface of the pan. Cook banana for 1 to 2 minutes until you start seeing a small amount of browning (caramelization) on the edges, then flip slices with a spatula, cooking for another couple of minutes. The banana slices will start melting and sticking together—this is OK.

3. Add the cooked brown rice to the pan and using the tip of the spatula, begin to mix rice with bananas, spreading the rice across the pan to ensure all the rice is thoroughly warmed. Cook another few minutes.

4. Add cinnamon and stir to combine. Remove, taste, and garnish the ceral with more cinnamon and add a small amount of milk if you wish and enjoy immediately!

Notes:

• Pasture-raised butter is butter that has been made from cows that have been grass-fed. If you cannot find grass-fed butter, use USDA organic.

• If you cook brown rice in advance, it can be stored in the refrigerator for several days and always comes in handy throughout the week as it is a great substitute for pasta and bread and accompanies all proteins, soups, stews and vegetable dishes brilliantly. Cooking brown rice is easiest in a rice cooker. I recommend investing in the rice cooker brand Zojirushi, which can be found at many retail outlets. Rice cookers can be used for oatmeal, white rice, and porridges.

Quinoa with Pinto Beans
with Avacado-Lime Dressing

This delicious recipe makes a great meatless dish, as the protein from the quinoa and healthy fat from the avocado dressing are wonderfully satisfying. This versatile dressing delivers salty, sweet, sour, and spicy all in one go!

SERVES: 4–6
TOTAL TIME: 30 MINUTES

INGREDIENTS FOR SALAD

- 1 c quinoa, rinsed and drained
- 1/2 tsp organic expeller pressed canola oil or olive oil or coconut oil
- 1/4–1/2 tsp ground cumin
- 1/2 tsp ground coriander
- 1/4 tsp chili powder
- 1/2 tsp sea salt
- 1 3/4 c filtered water
- 1 c organic pinto beans, rinsed several times, drained, and patted dry using paper towels
- 3/4 c red bell pepper, deseeded, membrane removed, cut into 1/4 inch pieces (about one small bell pepper)

INGREDIENTS FOR DRESSING

- 2 ripe organic avocados
- 5 tsp lime juice
- 3/8 tsp sea salt
- 1 1/2 inch piece serrano chili, deseeded, very finely minced
- 2 tsp coconut palm sugar or other WAMP sugar crystal (see page 59 for list)

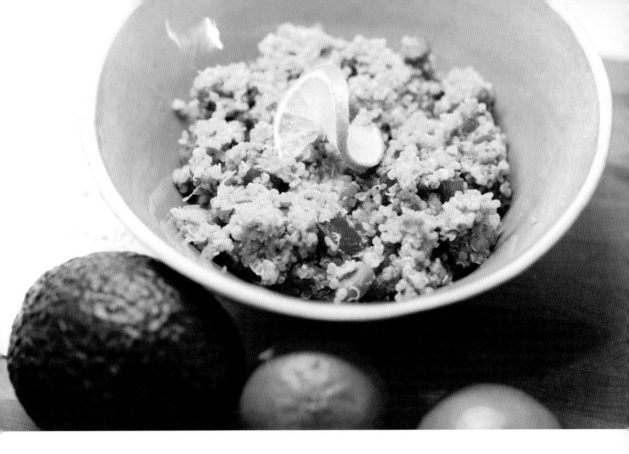

PROCEDURE

1. Place quinoa in a heavy saucepan, add oil, spices, and salt, and stir to combine over low heat. Add water, bring to a boil then lower to a simmer, cover, and cook for 20 minutes. Fluff with a fork, transfer quinoa to a large mixing bowl. Add pinto beans and bell peppers to quinoa, and gently stir to combine.

2. In a separate mixing bowl, mash avocados, adding lime juice simultaneously. Then add remaining ingredients and mash well to combine.

3. Transfer avocado dressing to quinoa mixing bowl and using a wooden spoon, gently stir to fully incorporate. Plate and serve!

Tabouli

WHEAT RESET RECIPE

Tabouli is a classic, centuries-old salad thought to have originated in Lebanon. Bulgur wheat is a great example of WAMP wheat, and in this dish, it is brought to life with a flavorful combination of fresh onions, tomatoes, mint, and parsley. Tabouli is guaranteed to awaken your taste buds and senses.

SERVES: 4–6
TOTAL TIME: 20 MINUTES

INGREDIENTS

- 1/3 c #1 bulgur (fine bulgur)
- 1/3 c boiling water
- 1 c small dice yellow or white onion (about 1 small onion)
- 1 c ripe tomato small dice (about 2 small tomatoes)
- 1 c (about 2 bunches) fresh mint leaves (discarding stems), rinsed thoroughly, dried (you may use paper towels) and chopped
- 2 bunches flat leaf parsley, using only leaves and discarding stems, rinsed and dried (you may use paper towels) chopped
- 4 tbsp lemon juice (about 2 lemons)
- 1/8 tsp ground pepper
- 1/4 tsp sea salt
- 2 tbsp extra-virgin olive oil
- 2 scallions, thinly sliced
- Several crisp romaine lettuce leaves (for plating)

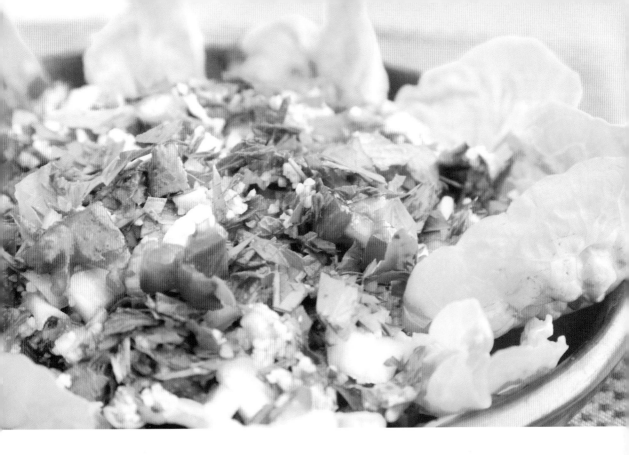

PROCEDURE

1. Place bulgur in bowl and poor boiling water overtop. Seal bowl with plastic wrap and set aside for 20 minutes, allowing bulgur to absorb water and fluff up.

2. When bulgur is ready, transfer to large mixing bowl. Add all remaining ingredients to the bowl with bulgur, taste for seasoning.

3. Plate tabouli over crisp romaine lettuce leaves, and enjoy!

Note: The two keys to making this recipe outstanding are the dryness of the greens—they should be as dry as possible—and tasting as you go. If you find at the end you need more acid/tang, add more lemon juice or a hint more salt whereas if you feel you could use more spiciness, add more scallion.

Dreamy Green Strawberry and Almond Smoothie

This easy to make smoothie is full of nourishing WAMP goodness, sweetened with dates, bananas, and strawberries. With homemade almond milk, it becomes even more luscious.

SERVES: 1
TOTAL TIME: 5 MINUTES

INGREDIENTS

- 5 frozen strawberries
- 3/8 c cold filtered water
- 1/4 c organic unsweetened apple juice (or coconut water)
- 1 c unsweetened almond milk
- 1 fresh date, pitted and halved
- 2 c fresh pre-washed baby spinach, patted down
- 1 ripe banana
- A few ice cubes (optional)

PROCEDURE

1. Place all ingredients into a blender and blend until creamy smooth.

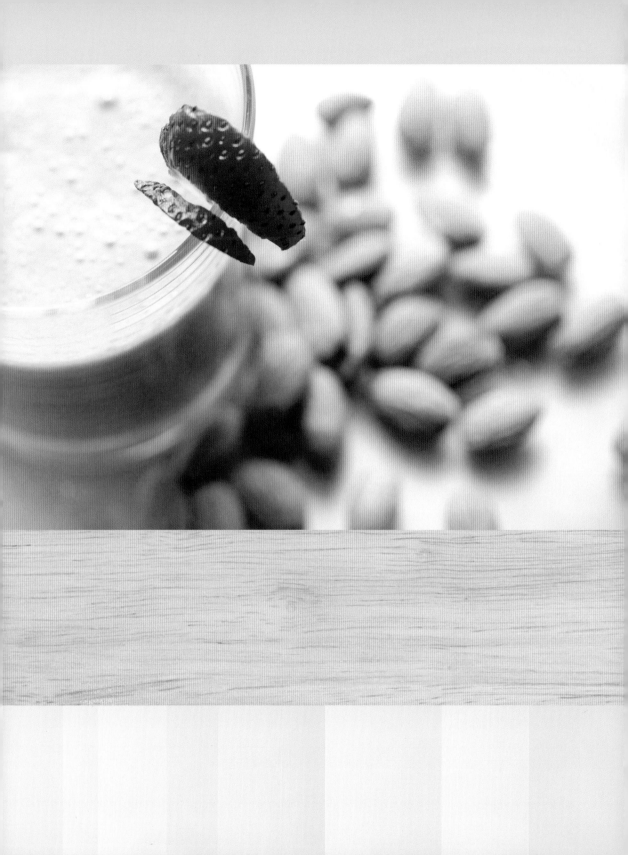

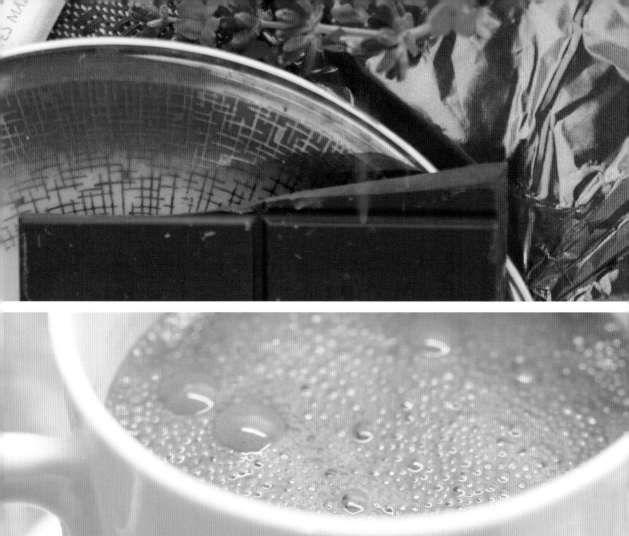
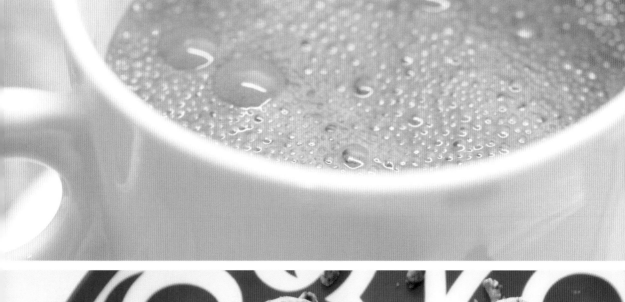

Chocolate
RESET

Ah, chocolate. When it comes to this brown, silky, creamy-smooth treat, we've got things all wrong, due to the simple fact that most of the chocolate we're eating isn't really chocolate in the first place.

Let me explain. Earlier in this book, I told you what a beautiful, naturally human thing it is to crave *healthy* food—WAMP food. Chocolate is no exception. In its WAMP form, chocolate is the ultimate guilt-free delight.

Except that the majority of commercially produced chocolate—the kisses, bunnies, coated nuts, cakes, and all that Halloween candy we've been so used to eating since we were old enough to go trick-or-treating—is far from the WAMP variety. Even the dark chocolate we've been told is the healthier kind may not be so good for you.

The reality is that most mass-produced chocolates are highly processed, watered-down versions of the real thing; they're so corrupted that in most instances they don't pass for chocolate in my book. The primary ingredients in mass-market chocolate aren't even brown.

Consuming this type of chocolate does us no favors. It doesn't nourish us, robs us of rich flavor, and leads to a relationship with chocolate that's severely dysfunctional. We need a chocolate reboot—desperately.

That's what this special Reset is all about—changing the way we know and enjoy chocolate in our daily lives. In this Reset we will completely redefine chocolate by learning about its origins, how it's made, and how much it has changed from its humble beginnings as a spicy drink revered by Mayan and Aztec royalty to a food that's too sweet, too light, and too ordinary for its own good.

In the end, our goal is to fall head over heels in love with a kind of chocolate that loves you back: an unadulterated, healthy, and delectable chocolate. After this reset, you'll be set on a path to enjoying chocolate that's better for you, and you'll stop being played by the processed, fake stuff once and for all. Let's get started!

Chocolate Isn't from Switzerland: What We Need to Know About Chocolate

Chocolate doesn't have its origins in Switzerland, or in Europe for that matter. Nor is chocolate an ingredient found in nature. Chocolate is in fact made up of a combination of *several ingredients*. You can think of chocolate as similar to bread, a food that's composed of four single ingredients: flour, yeast, water, and salt.

What gives chocolate its distinctive brown hue is the cacao seed (or bean), which comes from the bright yellow, maroon, and orange pods (also called fruit) of the cacao plant, a tree first cultivated in Central America around 1500 BC by ancient Mesoamerican civilizations, most notably the Mayans, who honored the tree as sacred. They called it *cacahuaquchtl*, a Mayan word for "tree."

Theobroma cacao (the tree's scientific name) is a relatively short, flowery plant that thrives in tropical forests shielded by other cash crops such as banana and rubber plants and other hardwood trees.

Each pod contains about fifty beans, which are surrounded by a white, sweet, soft pulp that is beloved by birds and monkeys. The beans are so bitter, however, that they're often discarded and left behind on the forest floor. Interestingly, the raw beans are not brown at first; they turn purple as they are first exposed to air. Cacao was so valuable that it was at times used as currency. The Mayans, one of the first peoples to make magic with cacao, didn't eat it; they drank it (supposedly gulped down in one swallow).

After harvesting the fruit and obtaining the beans, they left them to ferment, then roasted them, crushed them between stones, and mixed the resulting paste with hot water (cold water may also have been used), whisking it with twigs to create froth. Chili, musk, or honey may have been added, and then it was ready to drink. The Mayans called this drink *tchaca-houa*, and compared it to ambrosia (a divine food of the gods), which would bring immortality to those lucky enough to drink it. Vases used to serve and drink cacao beverages have been found that date back to AD 600. The Aztecs would later call the drink *tchocoatl*.

> Our goal is for you to fall head over heels in love with a kind of chocolate that loves you back—an unadulterated, nourishing, and delectable chocolate.

The Spanish would "discover" the drink in the sixteenth century, when conquistador Hernando Cortés overthrew the Aztec Empire in 1521. It is said that Cortés was offered the drink in fine golden cups by "delightfully unclad virgins," and that Montezuma, the ruler of the Aztecs, drank up to fifty cups of it per day.

At some point thereafter, by either an error in spelling or translation, or possibly from the Aztec word *xocolatl*, meaning "bitter water," the drink came to be called "chocolate."

Regardless of the name, it was in this way—as a spicy, bitter, and extremely minimally processed drink—that chocolate was savored for countless generations, making its way around the globe. The first shipment of cacao beans from Veracruz, Mexico, to Seville, Spain, took place in 1585. The beans and drink then made their way to Germany around the mid-1600s and became available only to the rich and elite, a luxury item as coveted as tea, sugar, and coffee. It's been recorded that a chocolate drink was served at a grand party at the palace of Versailles in 1682.

It wouldn't be until the nineteenth century that chocolate would be mass-produced in block form for eating as opposed to drinking. Mechanized milling, thanks in part to the Industrial Revolution and the invention of the steam engine, helped in this endeavor by allowing the extraction of cacao butter and better grinding capacities. Soon thereafter, chocolate became less expensive and more accessible to the masses. The first real chocolate factories opened in France around 1824.

From then on, the sacred, beloved, WAMP chocolate drink of the Mayans would be converted into a bevy of new forms and functions. After Swiss chemist Henri Nestlé invented powdered milk as a kind of infant formula, another Swiss, Daniel Peter, was able to use his methods to combine powdered milk and chocolate liqueur, ultimately inventing milk chocolate in 1876.

Back in America, in 1894 candy manufacturer Milton Hershey decided to add a chocolate coating to his caramels and opened the Hershey Chocolate Company.

Chocolate would never be the same again.

From "Drink of the Gods" to Processed Candy

Today, we're eating highly processed chocolate. In fact, there's not much *chocolate* in today's chocolate.

Here's how most commercial chocolate is made: After harvesting the cacao beans, they're usually fermented (traditionally in wooden boxes or in piles covered by banana leaves, although this step may get skipped altogether), dried, then roasted and crushed into what the industry describes as "nibs," which is basically chocolate in its purest form, its WAMP form. The nibs are then ground into a paste.

This mass is subjected to high-speed mills that generate sufficient heat to convert it into a thick liquid, what manufacturers refer to as "cacao liquor," also known as "cacao mass" (at this point, the liquid can be cooled to yield unsweetened baking chocolate or bitter chocolate).

After that, some of the liquid is further processed into two parts: "cocoa cake" (after milling it is sold as "cocoa powder"—what goes into things like cake mixes, syrups, and frostings and the stuff that gives chocolate all its flavor and its brown hue) and "cocoa butter." The separation is accomplished by using high-pressure milling technology (usually hydraulic pressure) to extract the cocoa butter from the liquor (cocoa butter has a pale yellow hue).

What happens next is the key turning point: a legion of other ingredients, usually ingredients that are themselves processed, join the manufacturing party. A specified amount of cacao liquor is mixed with cocoa butter as well as sugar—usually refined sugar. To this a bevy of fillers, usually processed, are added to make the solid chocolate bars and candy that line grocery stores aisles.

If it's milk chocolate the manufacturer is making, milk is added too. It may show up in a variety of forms—condensed, powdered, etc.—and is usually the factory-farmed variety. Next, lecithins (e.g., soy lecithin) are added to help bind the mixture. And finally, various additives, flavorings, and preservatives are mixed in to increase the taste intensity and prolong shelf life.

This concoction is then further ground in roller mills to convert it from a rough, granular mixture to a smooth, silky one. The process of "conching" furthers this transition by mixing, churning, swirling, and aerating the chocolate for several hours. Next, chocolate gets its trademark glossy sheen by way of "tempering," which happens by stirring the chocolate, letting it cool, heating it back up slowly, and repeating the process, and is then finally shaped it into molds, blocks, bars, chips, or left it in liquid form. All these products eventually make their way into Halloween treats, chocolate chip scones, tin-foil clad Easter bunnies, double chocolate cookies, M&M's, brownies, and powder dusted Valentine's truffles.

Very Little Chocolate

Unfortunately, with all the breaking apart, mixing, and modifying, this kind of chocolate product bears little resemblance to the ground nibs it originated from. Not only is it no longer a WAMP food, but it's been drowned out by ingredients that have not a smidgen to do with the *cacahuaquchtl* tree. These additional ingredients are so high in many end products that the cacao, which started off center stage, is now relegated to a behind-the-scenes role. What remains is very little cacao, if any.

Consider these eye-opening realities about how much cacao is really in chocolate. According to the FDA, "sweet chocolate" requires only 15 percent cocoa liquor; the remainder can be composed of sugars and other (usually) processed ingredients. "Semi-sweet" and "bittersweet" chocolate require only 35 percent. And "milk chocolate," the most popular type of chocolate and the kind that goes into Hershey's Kisses and Nestlé Crunch bars, doesn't have to have *any more than 10 percent cocoa liquor*. "White chocolate" contains only 20 percent cocoa butter, and it doesn't contain *any* brown cocoa liquor or solids.

Dark Chocolate

The FDA doesn't have a standard definition for "dark chocolate," which is chocolate that doesn't contain milk. These chocolates may contain very little cacao (e.g., 30 percent cacao) and don't need to specify anything to the buyer. In other words, if you buy a dark chocolate product, it doesn't necessarily mean you're about to eat a whole lot of healthy.

Chocolate-Flavored Sugar

Not surprisingly, the primary ingredient in most commercial chocolate is table sugar, not cacao. In effect, we're eating sugar *flavored* with chocolate.

Here's the ingredient label of a well-known milk chocolate bar. As you can see, sugar is the first ingredient on the list, which means it carries the most weight in the recipe.

Milk chocolate (**sugar**, cocoa butter, chocolate, lactose, skim milk, milk fat, soy lecithin, artificial flavor)

Here's the ingredient label of a well-known dark chocolate bar. As you can see, sugar is again at the top of the list.

Sugar, chocolate, cocoa butter, cocoa processed with alkali, milk fat, lactose, soy lecithin, PGPR, emulsifier, vanillin, artificial flavor, milk

It's time to get things straight: We're in love, but not with chocolate. What we're really eating is processed sugar seasoned with a smidgen of cacao.

The sad part is that we've lost our understanding of chocolate the way the Mayans made and enjoyed it, chock-full of nourishment: rich in protein, healthy fats, calcium, iron, carotene, thiamine, and riboflavin. This kind of WAMP chocolate (although it depends on how the chocolate was processed from bean to bar) is significantly rich in antioxidant flavanoids—the same stuff that gives green tea and red wine their health-promoting qualities.

Food Science Fillers and Flavorings

Cacao is bitter by itself. Even the rainforest animals know that, and favor the sweet pulp over the seeds. So, to round it out, the Mesoamerican peoples added a few WAMP ingredients, like spices and honey. They would be horrified if they knew what we're adding to it today. Food-science-concocted ingredients like palm kernel oil, corn syrup, HFCS, and lactose are now standard in many chocolates.

> We're in love, but not with chocolate—what we're really eating is processed sugar seasoned with a smidgen of cacao.

Take this name-brand dark chocolate truffle, for example—the kind of chocolate product that should be more authentic than the rest. The ingredient list does say it's made from chocolate (cocoa liquor), cocoa butter, and sugar, yet many other substances are also in tow: vegetable oil, condensed milk, soya lecithin, barley malt powder, and artificial flavors.

Bittersweet Chocolate (chocolate, sugar, cocoa butter, milk fat, soya lecithin, [emulsifier], vanilla seeds), **vegetable oil, (coconut, palm kernel)**, **sugar**, chocolate, cocoa butter, milk, **soya lecithin (emulsifier)**, **barley malt powder**, **artificial flavors**.

Nomenclature Fraud

We might do well to think of chocolate as we do perfume. Processed chocolate is similar to *eau de toilette*, in which a very small concentration of the true fragrances extracted from flowers and other fragrant substances is used, in contrast to *eau de parfum*. It's a watered-down product. Synthetic ingredients are used to fill in any gaps and keep costs low; it doesn't deliver the same potency, nor does it linger on the body as long. *Eau de toilettes* evaporate faster, they're cheaper, and their scents aren't as rich.

At least with perfumes, we're able to distinguish the inferior version from the superior version by the name on the package.

Cacao vs. Cocoa

Although the word "cocoa" is often used to describe a hot chocolate drink or the dry powder used to make hot chocolate, the term is more or less inter-changeable with "cacao."

But with chocolate, there are no such nomenclature distinctions. If I had it my way, there would be two completely different names for chocolate. Processed chocolate would be called "cocoa-flavored sugar butter" and WAMP chocolate would be rightly referred to as "chocolate." But alas, I'm not the FDA.

WAMP Chocolate

Now that we know about the pitfalls of processed chocolate, let's talk about the glori-ousness of real chocolate. I love teaching people about chocolate, especially how to find WAMP chocolate—something I've been doing with my clients and in my food writ-ing for years. When I first reset my own understanding of chocolate many years ago, I realized that I had been missing out for far too long. I'd been fooled by product labeling, advertising, and a false chocolate culture that had surrounded me since I was a tyke.

Although processed chocolate dominates our culinary landscape, there's plenty of WAMP chocolate out there—the healthier stuff that's in line with the Mayans' original recipes. You just have to know how and where to get your hands on it. Here are a few forms of WAMP chocolate you can savor:

Nibs

Cacao nibs, which are now sold today in many health food stores, are simply cacao beans shelled and cut up into pieces. They're hard and deliciously bitter—lovely in cereals, frozen yogurts, and just about anywhere you're looking for a crunch.

If you can get your hands on nibs, these are the best representation of the beans the Mayans used along with water and spices to make *tchocoatl* a millennia ago. If you wanted

> ## Cacao Liquor
>
> According to the National Confectioners Association's Chocolate Council, cacao liquor may also be described as "chocolate liquor," "cocoa solids," "cocoa mass," "cacao mass," or simply "chocolate."

to, you could pulverize these nibs into a paste, add boiling water and honey, and you'd have *tchocoatl* in the comfort of your own home.

And of course, because nibs are simply the whole beans cut up, they are the definition of "whole food and minimally processed food"—WAMP food. That means they're wonderfully nourishing. Whole cacao beans have been found to be high in flavonoids and other vitamins and minerals such as magnesium, and even fiber.

Cacao Powder

Many companies now offer cacao powder that can be used in baking and to make hot chocolate and countless other chocolate-flavored foods and drinks.

Although cacao powder is not a whole food—it consists of the beans ground into a paste, the butter extracted, and the remaining solids milled into a light powder—it's minimally processed.

The Super WAMP version of cacao powder is raw cacao powder. This powder is made by ensuring that the cacao isn't exposed to high temperatures (which kill off many nutrients)—usually what the industry refers to as "cold milling." Many companies providing raw powder also use organic beans.

When you're looking for this type of WAMP chocolate, there should be a single ingredient on the ingredient list: "cacao powder." That's it.

WAMP Chocolate Bars

Next and last is WAMP chocolate in the form of solid bars. This is the kind of solid chocolate that's simply made and delicious: true, healthy, dark chocolate.

WAMP bars can come with just two ingredients: cocoa beans and sugar. However, more often you'll see three. The ingredient lists on these products may look something like this:

Ingredients: Cocoa beans (or cocoa liquor), cocoa butter, sugar

The ordering of those three ingredients is key. Notice that WAMP chocolate bars are made primarily of cacao, so that will always be the *first* ingredient on any WAMP chocolate bar ingredient list.

Now, if you want to have a WAMP chocolate bar with a bit of extra flavoring, you can find many that are made of delightful WAMP ingredients such as vanilla beans, coconut, and mint. This of course, will get us up to four ingredients:

Ingredients: Cocoa beans (or cocoa liquor), cocoa
butter, sugar, ground vanilla beans

Pay special attention to the percentage of cacao in a bar. Even though cacao may be first on the list, we also need to make sure there's *a lot* of it. The more cacao in the bar, the closer the bar is to the chocolate the Aztecs ate. I like to define WAMP chocolate as having at least 70 percent cacao. You'll see the amount of cacao featured on the front of all WAMP chocolate bars, usually stated as "% cacao," which represents the total percentage of ingredients by weight in that product that come from the cocoa bean (i.e., chocolate liquor and cocoa butter).

If you don't see a percentage of cacao featured on the front of the package, don't buy it, because it's likely not WAMP!

Unbelievable Flavor

Just as the majority of us have never had the opportunity to taste real sugarcane or real wheat berries, we've never had a shot at experiencing the true flavor of chocolate.

The flavor of pure cacao ("flavor" defined by both taste and smell) is magically nuanced and complex. There's not just one note. Cacao, and the WAMP chocolate

Four Ingredients. That's All.

WAMP bars can be identified by taking a look at the ingredient list on the packaging. The list should have no more than these four ingredients:

- Cocoa liquor or cocoa beans (may also read as "cocoa solids" or "cocoa mass")
- Sugar (preferably a WAMP sugar)
- Cocoa butter
- Additional flavor ingredient, such as mint or vanilla beans

products it's made into, can be described as "fruity," "floral," "butterscotch," "coffee," "spicy," or even "musky."

In fact, WAMP chocolate has more flavor compounds than wine, the cacao bean naturally containing almost 1,500 flavors alone. Just as we do wine tastings, we can do chocolate tastings too, as many experts do.

There are myriad interesting factors at play that dictate the flavor in WAMP chocolate. Terroir—the environment where specific cacao beans come from (particularly soil, geography, plant variety, and climate)—can make a certain WAMP chocolate bar taste more fruity than another, for example. Chocolate based on beans from Ecuador will taste different from chocolate made from beans harvested in Madagascar.

Chocolate flavor also comes from the fermentation and roasting processes, the length and methodology both affecting aroma and flavor. The conching process also dictates flavor. WAMP chocolate is a far more sophisticated, nuanced, and flavorful chocolate than anything you'll ever find in commercial, sugar-packed chocolate, so don't settle for junk when you can have a jewel.

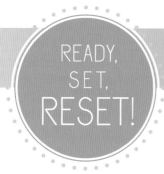

READY, SET, RESET!

In this Reset, the way you experience chocolate will forever be changed. Now, I ask you to put everything you now know about chocolate into action!

To fully appreciate WAMP chocolate, you will put all your senses to work: touching, smelling, seeing, and tasting it.

It's only when we're able to partake of food in a physical sense that we're able to have the chance to fall in love with it, and make the necessary healthy transitions we desperately want to make.

Instructions

Over a three-day period, eat only from the Reset recipes below, substituting these daily chocolate tastings for all your daily desserts or sweet foods, so your taste buds can fully acclimate to pure chocolate and not get confused by other sugary treats.

You can start with any recipe you'd like and don't necessarily have to eat all three recipes over the three days. Of course, if you do, you'll have a better understanding of WAMP chocolate when you're done.

Because WAMP chocolate has much less sugar than processed, commercial chocolate, these new recipes may not satiate every sweet tooth. If that's the case, feel free to also use the recipes from the Sugar Reset chapter to help support you as you go along, one recipe per day.

To purchase nibs and cacao powder, you may want to seek out a natural foods grocer in your community. Although some of these items may seem relatively pricey, please keep in mind that healthy chocolate—the kind we all want to be eating—can't compete with the unhealthy, processed variety on prices because it can't cut corners in the way it's made.

The Dark Side of Cacao

WAMP chocolate is delicious and healthy, but I would be remiss not to mention a darker side that comes with its production—something we should keep at the top of our minds when resetting our relationship with this modern-day ambrosia.

Cacao pods need to be harvested from trees, cut open, and fermented before they complete their transformation from bean to bar. Unfortunately, in some countries such as Côte d'Ivoire, which produces 40 percent of the world's cacao beans (70 percent of beans come from West Africa alone), these tasks are the domain of children as young as ten years of age who are enslaved or trafficked across borders. UNICEF estimates that nearly a half million children work on farms across the Ivory Coast, "engaged in the worst forms of child labor."

> WAMP chocolate is far more sophisticated, nuanced, and flavorful than anything you'll ever find in commercial, sugar-packed chocolate, so don't settle for junk when you can have a jewel.

Cacao production also taxes the environment and our vital rainforests. As demand for chocolate has risen, cacao-farming operations have opted to destroy an untold amount of rainforest to grow cacao more intensively, thereby disrupting the fragile ecosystems that are maintained when it is cultivated the way Mother Nature intended.

With this destruction not only are agrochemicals used where they were previously unnecessary, but these chemicals contaminate the water supply and erode soil health. And countless threatened plant and animal species fall at risk—species we depend on for the health of natural evolutionary processes and for the health of our planet.

Rebooting our chocolate fix requires that we keep both the above in mind. To ensure we are consuming chocolate that's both socially and environmentally responsible, choose chocolate that is certified IMO Fair for Life and USDA Organic.

TIPS & TOOLS for EACH DAY

Day One

You're here. Welcome to your first day of experiencing chocolate anew!

On this first day, start by making a simple mental adjustment. Decide that today you will make a conscious effort to focus on the chocolate products that surround you every day—something you may never have thought to do before this Reset.

Since you'll be forgoing your usual treats for your new WAMP chocolate ones, take a moment to examine them today: Do the cookies you usually eat after lunch have chocolate in them? If so, what kind of chocolate? What is included on the ingredient list? How about the chocolate fudge or chips in your favorite ice cream? What kind of chocolate is in them? Investigate. Realize just how much chocolate surrounds you each and every day without you even knowing.

To keep things simple on this first day, you may want to start off with the first recipe—WAMP chocolate squares. This kind of solid WAMP chocolate is already made for you so today you don't have to do anything at all except break a square off your bar and eat.

Solid WAMP chocolate like this is easy to carry with you. You can throw it in your lunch sack or purse.

Take a bite of your chocolate when you want to have a bit of sweetness. Today this might happen right after you finish your lunch, or maybe in midafternoon when you're feeling like you need a pick-me-up.

One thing you may want to keep in mind with this kind of WAMP chocolate is that you don't want to pop a square in your mouth and swallow. You want to take your time.

A lot of the flavor you will experience with WAMP chocolate comes from what industry experts call "mouthfeel." When eating your chocolate square, make sure you take small bites at a time, and pause for a moment letting the chocolate linger on your tongue, feeling its texture and richness. As you eat it, also take a moment to reflect on its aroma and the flavor notes you're sensing. Does this chocolate taste nutty or fruity? Does it seem bolder than chocolate you're used to?

Realize that this kind of chocolate will taste different because it has much more cacao, less milk, less sugar, and no processed ingredients.

Notice, too, how much more satisfied you feel with this kind of chocolate, even though you're eating such a small amount. Do you want to have another square, or do you feel satiated? For most people, this kind of chocolate is more rewarding and curbs cravings because it has a higher percentage of cacao butter and less craving-inducing refined sugar.

As you move along into the evening, maybe make it a point to share your new chocolate journey with friends or colleagues. Let them know what you're doing for the next three days with chocolate and ask them what they know about it. Do they realize how much sugar is in most commercial chocolate? Do they realize that they're likely not tasting the true flavor of real cacao? Do they know that most chocolate is milk chocolate, the kind that was invented only about 150 years ago?

If you decide to finish off the day with another square of chocolate—perhaps after dinner this evening—take one last moment to opine on this new version of chocolate you're experiencing. If you find it 180 degrees opposite to the chocolate you're used to, that's OK! That's what you're supposed to sense. Don't resist the fact that WAMP chocolate isn't at all similar to processed chocolate. Just welcome this new understanding into your life and reward yourself for expanding your palate. Congratulations on finishing your first day!

Day Two

Good morning! Today you may want to consider making the hot chocolate. This recipe is a great one because this kind of beverage will make you rethink what you have understood to be "hot chocolate" most of your life.

You may opt to make this drink at any time today—maybe after lunch, or when your kids come home from school, or as a before-bed treat.

When taking your first sips, think about how much more cacao flavor you taste versus sugar flavor and sweetness. Compare this kind of drink with the hot chocolate you make either by combining boiling water with one of those single pouches of hot chocolate powder mix or by mixing milk with a chocolate syrup.

> For most people, this kind of chocolate is more rewarding and curbs cravings because it has a higher percentage of cacao butter and less craving-inducing refined sugar

Also note how much richer, deeper, and more complex this kind of drink is compared to the processed versions. Examine the label of the cacao powder you've purchased. Realize how little fat is in this powder, as the cacao butter has been extracted.

If you decide you don't want to make hot chocolate or don't have the time and would rather continue eating the chocolate squares today, that's OK too.

Regardless of what you choose, as you go about your business today, continue to keep your eyes open to where processed chocolate hides. You'll realize that it seems to be everywhere: granola bars, cereal, candy coating, chocolate-coated nuts, baked goods, biscotti, scones, etc.

Day Three

Today is your final day of experiencing healthier, better chocolate. On this day, try out the final recipe, the fabulous WAMP chocolate truffles! After assembling your ingredients, this recipe should take you no more than five minutes from start to finish. It's a must-do if you have the time, as it allows you to taste cacao nibs—which are one of the most whole forms of cacao on the planet. Tasting nibs will help you understand what the Mayans, Aztecs, and most of Europe (prior to the seventeenth century) tasted when they indulged in chocolate hundreds of years ago.

If today is a workday for you, you may opt to take along a square or two of chocolate for the day and when you come home, make the truffles.

As you're making the truffles, try to eat just the nibs—maybe about a teaspoon worth. How does it taste? Instead of sweet, you're likely finding bitter, right? How about the texture? And color? Take time here to really feel, see, and taste the nibs before you put them in the blender.

When you're finally ready to try your truffles, remember to take small bites because when you're using WAMP cacao powder and nibs, you're getting much more fiber and fat—both of which tend to satisfy you faster and easier. You're also getting a lot more richness and depth of flavor with smaller portions.

Finish off this last day by reflecting on what you've learned in the last seventy-two hours. How has your definition of chocolate changed? What have your taste buds experienced? Share your story and your new relationship with chocolate with others.

After the Reset

Bravo! Now that you've completed this important Reset, your relationship with chocolate has likely been entirely reprogrammed. Over the last three days you've had the opportunity—possibly for the first time in your life—to experience gloriously rich chocolate flavor that isn't masked by sugar, milk, or other additives. You became aware of all the mountains of fake chocolate products that surround you daily—products you grew up thinking were chocolate, but really aren't. You've experienced chocolate that's more satisfying and rewarding. You now know that WAMP chocolate is something fundamentally different from both a flavor and a health perspective. It's this kind of chocolate that we're meant to crave!

You also now have a set of skills to help you detect and shop for WAMP chocolate and you won't fall prey to food-marketing gimmicks or trends. You'll know that even though that dark chocolate–covered graham cracker may be marketed as healthier for you, unless it gives you a "% cacao" on the label, it's likely processed chocolate. You'll finally be in control when you walk down the chocolate aisle. Don't be surprised if your friends start calling you a "chocolate snob."

Although most people fall in love with WAMP chocolate, particularly the solid bars, if you didn't during these three days, that's OK. The flavor of WAMP chocolate is fundamentally unique and different. But just know that the chocolate you may like instead is more sugar and milk than cacao.

But if you're interested in furthering your health by eating more whole and minimally processed foods (as I'm sure you are—you're reading this book!), don't give up so fast. For some people, it takes time to adjust to WAMP chocolate, especially if your taste buds are so used to the high amount of sugar in processed foods.

Try following my 80/20 Rule to keep you on this path as you leave this chapter.

YOUR CHOCOLATE RESET GROCERY LIST

- ☐ Chocolate bar, 70 percent or greater cacao
- ☐ Unsweetened almond milk, another nut milk, or organic and/or grass-fed whole or 2 percent milk
- ☐ Unsweetened cacao powder
- ☐ Pure maple syrup
- ☐ 1/2 lb raw pecans
- ☐ 1/2 lb Medjool or Deglet Noor dates, seeds removed, roughly chopped
- ☐ Cacao nibs
- ☐ 1 package fresh raspberries

Keep in mind that over time, if you follow this rule, you may find that you start to like WAMP chocolate more and more, and processed chocolate may give you headaches or taste too harsh for your liking. Over time, don't be surprised if you find yourself taking a pass on all those Easter and holiday chocolates. They'll just be too sweet to taste good to you!

One final tip: As you move on from this Reset and want to find more WAMP chocolate products to indulge in, a good rule of thumb to follow is if a product doesn't come with an ingredient list—even if it looks dark and of high quality—and you can't figure out what's in it (even by asking a sales clerk), it's best to pass.

70 Percent+ Cacao Chocolate Square

CHOCOLATE RESET RECIPE

Have a 1 1/2-inch square piece of a 70 percent cacao (or higher), solid chocolate bar as your dessert, up to twice per day. Read the ingredients list and make sure the below apply:

- Cacao must be the first ingredient.
- There should be no more than three to four ingredients which may include:
    1. Cacao beans (or cacao solids or cacao butter)
    2. Sugar
    3. Cocoa butter
    4. A flavoring ingredient (e.g., mint, fruit, nuts, etc.)
- Milk (in any form) must not be listed.

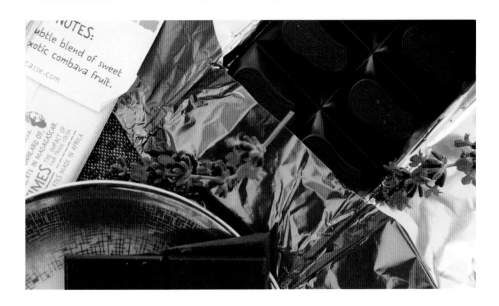

Basic Hot Chocolate

This WAMP hot chocolate is satisfying and dreamy, and can be made in a snap. You'll immediately realize that this hot chocolate outclasses all the rest.

SERVES: 1
TOTAL TIME: 5 MINUTES

INGREDIENTS

- 1 c unsweetened almond milk, another nut milk, or organic and/or grass-fed whole or 2% milk
- 2 tbsp pure, unsweetened cacao powder or 1 1/2 inch square piece of a WAMP chocolate bar
- 2 tsp (or to taste) pure maple syrup

PROCEDURE

1. In a heavy-bottomed, small saucepan, heat almond milk over low-medium heat.

2. Turn heat to low, add cocoa or chocolate square and syrup, and gently mix together using a small whisk. Whisk until fully incorporated and slightly frothy. Pour into a cup and enjoy hot.

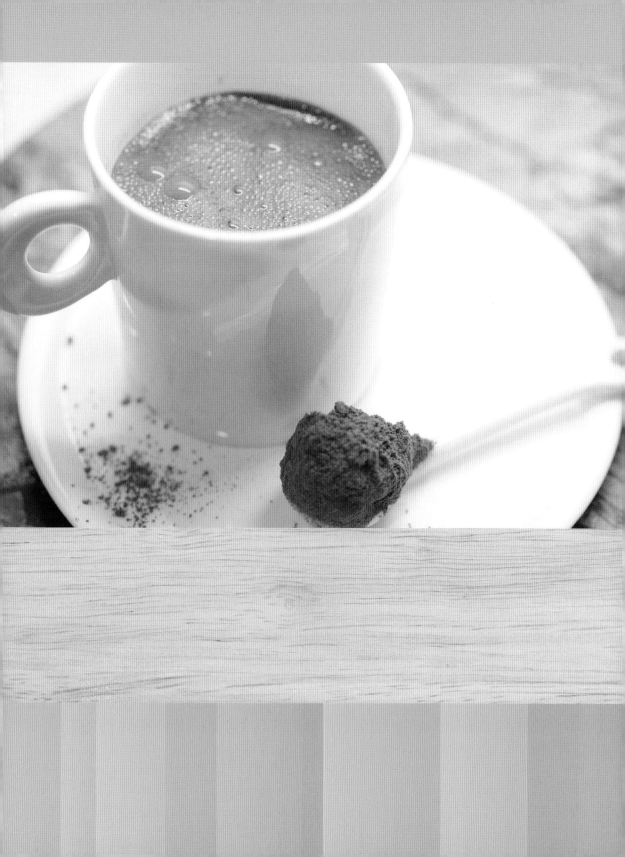

Raspberry Chocolate Truffles

Two ancient ingredients—cacao and dates—maake this WAMP recipe perfect for vital living. Combined with ripe raspberries, these truffles are the perfect companion to a hot cup of coffee or tea.

SERVES: 16 TRUFFLES
TOTAL TIME: 10 MINUTES

INGREDIENTS

- 1 c raw pecans
- 1 c Medjool or Deglet Noor dates, seeds removed, roughly chopped
- 2 tbsp unsweetened cacao powder (raw if possible), plus extra for dusting
- 2 tbsp cacao nibs
- 1/4 c fresh raspberries

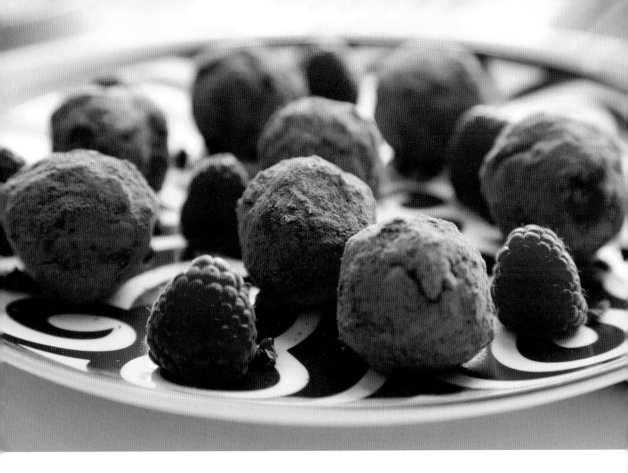

PROCEDURE

1. Pour a small amount of cacao powder onto a sheet or large plate for coating and dusting the truffles.

2. Add all ingredients to a food processor or blender, and blend until ingredients are fully incorporated and pecans and dates are chopped into small bits. Be careful not to overblend. If the mixture looks too dry, add a couple of extra raspberries.

3. Scoop out the truffle mixture using a tablespoon. Scoop 1 1/2 tablespoons at a time, forming each into a ball with your hands. Transfer balls to dusting plate and coat thoroughly, then tap the truffle to remove any excess powder.

4. Enjoy immediately with tea or coffee or chill in the refrigerator for an hour or more. Truffles will last in the fridge for several days.

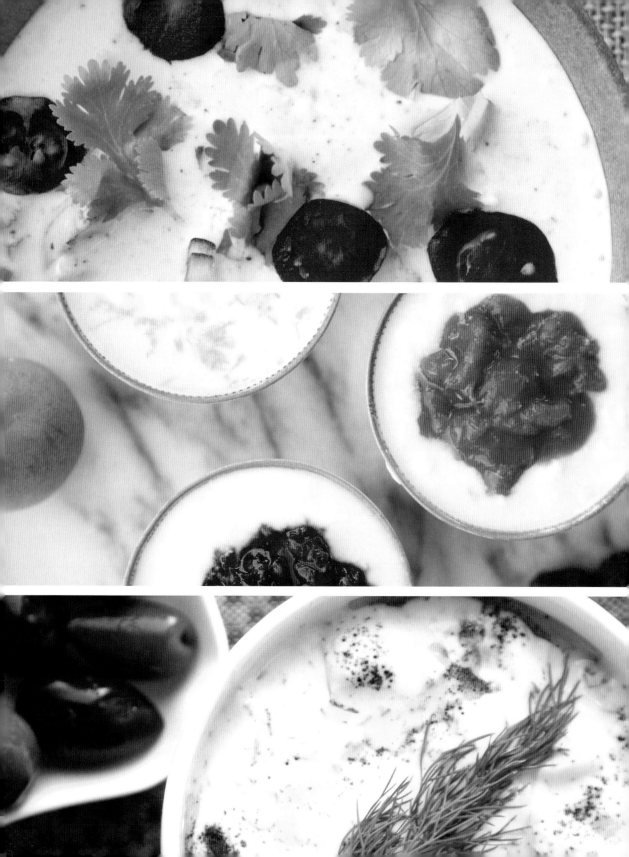

Yogurt
RESET

Yogurt has one of the most successful gigs in all the food biz. It's like a Celine Dion contract at Caesars Palace in Vegas—worth megamillions. Except, unlike Celine, yogurt didn't earn its spot fair and square. Let me explain.

Today's average grocery-store yogurt claims to be the ultimate health food: convenient and deliciously "light and fluffy"; full of probiotics; high in calcium, protein, and vitamin D; and available in an array of fun-filled flavors from Mixed Berry to Boston Cream Pie—the perfect go-to food for kids and adults who want to live a fit and active lifestyle.

Unfortunately, all these claims are nothing more than a bunch of hot air. Today's commercial yogurts are nothing more than processed, sugary imposters of authentic, WAMP yogurt. They're poseurs.

Modern yogurt is a fake "healthy food," propelled by an ingenious marketing ploy that makes us believe we're eating healthily when we're really not.

Our current relationship with yogurt is radically off-course. But it's no fault of our own. Fake yogurt is everywhere, and it comes in every shape, size, texture, name, and function that we can't help but be attracted to it. In Yogurtland, there's a permutation to meet your every need and desire: low-fat, extra-creamy, whipped, granola-topped, and "fruit on the bottom." The Yoplait brand itself offers nearly forty flavors: everything from "Pineapple Upside-Down Cake" to "Twisted Screamin' Green Apple." There's set yogurt, blended yogurt, and yogurts that help support the gut with "10 billion probiotic cultures."

All of this is a distraction from WAMP yogurt, the kind that we *should* be craving, yogurt that is pure, honest, and utterly delicious. This Reset fixes what's broken.

Food of the Gods: What We Need to Know About Yogurt

It's lusciously smooth, we eat it cold, and we know that it fits somewhere between eggs and cream cheese in the dairy aisle, but what exactly *is* yogurt?

Put simply, yogurt is fermented milk. Although no one knows exactly how yogurt was first invented in human history, it likely happened thousands of years ago, with milk coming into contact with wild bacteria cultures in the air. Bacteria ferment natural sugars in milk called lactose, and produce lactic acid, which then interacts with proteins in the milk, transforming it into the white, creamy creation we call yogurt.

Pastoral, nomadic tribes were likely the first benefactors of this luscious delight simply because of their ease of access to ruminants like sheep and yak that they traveled with. History suggests that yogurt put down strong roots with the people of the Balkans—the southeastern region of Europe, particularly Bulgaria, is referred to as the "cradle of yogurt." However, some records suggest that it was consumed by the people of Iran and India since ancient times.

Why was it such a hit way back when? History suggests it most likely had to do with its health properties. You see, when milk gets a chance to ferment, it transforms into a food that contains a large amount of bacteria—not the icky, make-you-sick stuff, but the kind of friendly bacteria we really want and need. Yogurt's bacteria support our digestive system by cultivating the "beneficial" bacteria in our bodies—and that's the bacteria that help cure digestive ailments and allergies, strengthen our bodies' defenses, and even increase longevity—a finding by Nobel Prize–winning Russian scientist Ilya Mechnikov in the early 1900s.

This feature has helped yogurt and its fermented brethren—kefir, koumiss, and curdled milk—stand the test of time. The venerable Mongol warlord Genghis Khan purportedly offered yogurt to his army to keep them strong. It's been well documented that in the sixteenth century, when King François I of France had a nasty case of diarrhea, he summoned a doctor from Turkey to bring him yogurt. That doctor walked the entire journey on foot with his herd of sheep to administer this "medicine."

Still, yogurt would continue to be a little-known, homemade recipe passed down by grandmas until as late as the twentieth century. That's when, prompted by discoveries at the Institut Pasteur in France, yogurt would finally make its global debut. A doctor by the name of Isaac Carasso, a Greek native with family ties to the Ottoman Empire, learned of the invention at the Institut of pure isolated bacteria strains that could mimic cultures found in nature. He realized that the healthful yogurt his ancestors made could now be duplicated and manufactured in factories on a large scale. In 1919, he set up shop in Spain and called his company Danone, originally selling yogurt to pharmacies in the way it had historically been used—as a medicinal product. It was marketed as "a traditional Bulgarian preparation assuring a long and healthy life."

> Fake yogurt not only is everywhere but comes in every shape, size, texture, name, and function that we can't help but be attracted to it.

Carasso eventually moved his operations to France, and in 1947 introduced something that would significantly change its trajectory: the inclusion of fruit jam, which not only made yogurt more palatable to sugar-craving Western tastes, boosting its popularity, but also conveniently helped prevent spoilage. With the preservation qualities of sugar in tow, yogurt could now be transported and stored for longer—a boon for business. The company began operations in the United States in 1942 under the name Dannon.

Although slow to take off in America—embraced only among the counterculture, Flower Power generation of the 1960s as an edgy health food—by the late twentieth century, yogurt had become a wildly popular, mainstream staple on grocery lists. Even the USDA found it tough to ignore, finally adding yogurt to its "annual book of dairy statistics"—but not until 1989.

Over the last thirty years, per capita yogurt consumption has increased a shocking 400 percent—the most profitable, fastest-growing segment in all the dairy industry. Today, industrially crafted yogurt has taken over the dairy aisle with countless offshoots and permutations, from drinkable smoothies and probiotic shots to Greek yogurts and yogurts mixed with high-fiber cereal. In fact, Greek yogurt has become so dominant that members of Congress have requested that the Secretary of Agriculture to modify USDA guidelines to include it as a source of protein, right up there with cheese and eggs.

Fraudster

Unfortunately, we have some waking up to do when it comes to modern yogurt. Although Carasso planted the seeds for yogurt to go viral, in the process it went from being one of humankind's first WAMP foods to one of the most processed dairy foods on the market.

The yogurt we're consuming today is not the same stuff King François I ate, or the food of ancient Persia, or the treasured recipes passed down by generations of Bulgarian grandmothers. The majority of the neatly stacked, colorfully branded peel-back cups you see today has been corrupted.

It's Not Supposed to Be Sweet!

Most of the resetting we need to do with yogurt has to do with taste. Ready for this? *Yogurt is not supposed to taste sweet.* Yogurt was never intended to taste like pineapples or strawberries. You were never meant to stick your spoon all the way down to the bottom of the cup expecting to find something sweet at the bottom. Adding fresh fruit to WAMP yogurt can be terrific, yes. But mixing in sugary processed fruit, table-sugar-spiked jam, or a food-science concoction that brags of its sweet "natural flavor" is not. It may taste pleasant, but so do candy, soda, and all kinds of foods we avoid because they aren't good for us.

Real yogurt, true yogurt, is *sour*—the polar opposite of how we're used to tasting it in America and most of the Western world. Yes, it's smooth, firm, and custard-like in texture, just like those store-bought brands. But the healthiest, WAMP yogurt tastes acidic, tangy, and tart. It's another kind of delicious!

Adding refined sugar to yogurt is a practice yogurt manufacturers use to help extend its shelf life. We know what refined sugar does: The more we eat it, the more our palate gets used to exaggerated levels of it, and the more we stop liking naturally sweet, WAMP foods. Which is exactly what happens when we taste plain, minimally processed yogurt for the very first time. "It tastes wrong," we complain. "It tastes *way too sour*!" In reality, yogurt isn't as acidic as it may seem—it's just that when juxtaposed to all that sweetness, our taste buds can't register its deliciousness in the right way.

> In reality, yogurt isn't as acidic as it may seem—it's just that juxtaposed to all that sweet, our taste buds can't register its tangy goodness in the right way.

We may be accustomed to the sweet stuff, but the natural sourness in yogurt is a beautiful thing and has been relished for millennia. Throughout most of its existence in our culinary history, yogurt has been eaten in ways that have absolutely zilch to do with sugar. My father, who spent his entire childhood in India, remembers how he and my grandfather drank a fresh, homemade yogurt drink called matta every morning. Spiced with cumin, pepper, and curry leaves, it was a daily delicacy.

Both the Indians and the Greeks made tangy, sour, soup-like concoctions of yogurt with onions, cucumbers, garlic, and herbs—the Indian version called raita, and the Greek, tzatziki. Persians and Indians also use yogurt for tenderizing meat, poultry, and fowl in such world-famous dishes as tandoori chicken and shish kebabs.

Extreme Processing

Not only has food processing changed the flavor profile of yogurt, it has completely dismantled its original recipe.

Yogurt in its WAMP state is made with just two basic ingredients: milk (from a sheep, goat, cow, etc.) and wild bacteria (or man-made bacteria strains called *Streptococcus thermophilus* and *Lactobacillus bulgaricus*).

The ingredient lists on today's processed yogurts look nothing like this. You'll still see "milk" (although now it can be non-fat or low-fat, as well as whole) and "bacteria," but there's also a whole slew of extra ingredients, and some peculiar ones at that. Locust bean gum, anyone? Potassium sorbate? How about some Yellow #6, and whey mineral complex?

On a recent visit to my neighborhood supermarket, I found an unbelievable array of ingredients in the yogurt aisle, as seen in the table at right.

Armed with the understanding of our weakness for sugar and our desire for a "melt away" mouthfeel, many yogurt companies have taken extreme processing measures to concoct the "perfect" yogurt for us that also maximizes sales.

Thickeners like modified cornstarch, agar, guar gum, and milk solids help impart just the right amount of creaminess. Stabilizers improve mouthfeel. Refined sweeteners like fruit juice concentrates satisfy our addiction to sweetness, while "natural flavorings" provide the perfect tool for concocting any imaginable flavor, from cotton candy to black forest cake.

Today's Yogurt: Fake Dessert

I remember how mesmerized I was by the yogurt aisle when I was a kid. Although my mom wasn't a big fan of bringing those peel back six-ounce cups of yogurt into the house (likely because of the high price tag), I keenly recall how they all sounded so alluring: key lime pie, strawberry-banana, maple vanilla.

I was curious to see just how much things have changed, so on a recent jaunt to my neighborhood grocery store I set aside some time to really investigate. I was shocked! The once simple menu of flavor options had become a full-blown kaleidoscope of choices.

The mainstay flavors of my youth were still alive and kickin', but now seemed run-of-the-mill in comparison with their new competition. The exotic had taken over: mango, pomegranate, pineapple-coconut. In addition to key lime pie, there was Boston cream pie, white chocolate raspberry, and titles you wouldn't be surprised to find on the dessert menu of five-star restaurants.

The flavor of these products wouldn't be possible without the help of food scientists. Professional flavorists clothed in white lab coats and armed with droppers have made cheesecake and caramel toffee flavorings possible.

Ingredients in WAMP Yogurt

- Raw or pasteurized milk

- Wild or human-made bacteria cultures

Ingredients in Processed Yogurt

- *L. Acidophilus*
- *Bifidus*
- Grade A pasteurized milk
- Vanilla-flavored syrup
- Corn starch
- Cherry juice concentrate
- Fruit juice (for color)
- Vegetable juice (for color)
- Carob bean gum
- Potassium sorbate
- Tricalcium phosphate
- Modified food starch
- Inulin
- Acacia gum
- Carmine (for color)
- Sodium citrate
- Sucralose
- Calcium lactate
- Acesulfame potassium
- Malic acid
- Xantham gum
- Sugar
- Water
- Natural flavor
- Pectin
- Locust bean gum
- Lemon juice concentrate
- Asparatame
- Red #40
- Turmeric extract
- HFCS
- Dextrose
- Blue #1
- Yellow #6
- Chocolate liquor
- Caramel color
- Agar
- Whey mineral complex
- Milk solids

So not only is yogurt similar to dessert, it's a synthetic dessert. Yogurt manufacturers have taken a simple, wildly healthful, ancient food and turned it into an unnecessarily complex, nutrient-defective, dumbed-down excuse for eating.

Craving WAMP Yogurt

Now lets turn our attention to craving WAMP yogurt, the healthiest, most delicious kind of yogurt there is. This kind of yogurt tastes marvelously cooling, sumptuously rich,

Buyer Beware! Health Claims Under Fire

Newly invented, patented, super-secret strains of isolated bacteria cultures are now showing up in yogurts and yogurt drinks the world over, promising to help boost immunity and support your healthy, active, on-the-go lifestyle. Dannon's DanActive now boasts *L. Casei immunitas* and Activa, *Bifidus regularis*, otherwise known as ActivaBifidobacterium lactis DN-173 010. Yet no research has conclusively shown their claims to be true. In Europe, the European Food Safety Authority slapped Dannon for unsubstantiated claims for its Activia products in 2010, and in a separate scandal, resulting in a lawsuit in the United States, Dannon had to pony up $35 million on the back of similar charges.

and distinctly tart and tangy. Plain WAMP yogurt is truly a beautiful addition to our culinary landscape.

As we learned earlier, the best yogurt on the planet has just two basic ingredients: milk (whether from sheep, cows, or goats) and bacteria cultures *Streptococcus thermophilus* and *Lactobacillus bulgaricus*. Obviously, the better quality your milk—sustainably sourced, from grass-fed animals—the tastier your yogurt will be. So when you're at the supermarket, read the labels closely to make sure you're choosing the highest quality, least processed plain yogurt around.

Perfect Pairings: How to Eat WAMP Yogurt

One of the biggest mishaps in our current relationship with yogurt, particularly in the Western world, is the manner in which we consume it. Yogurt wasn't meant to be eaten as a solo dish or a snack. Yogurt was never meant to be eaten by itself out of a plastic, peel-back container.

Instead, yogurt is best as a *complement* to main dishes. For hundreds of years, dozens of cultures have dressed plain yogurt with a variety of herbs, spices, and vegetables to consume it as a drink, soup, condiment, marinade, or dip.

Yogurt forms the base of some of the most famous dishes the world over, from

Frozen Yogurt: "Healthy" Is Hype

Fro yo fans: I'm sorry to say it, but frozen yogurt is nothing more than an ice-cold processed dessert and another ingenious way of marketing a treat as "healthy" when it's not.

Frozen yogurt was invented in 1971 when an employee of the HP Hood dairy company sent regular yogurt through a soft-serve ice cream machine. It quickly gained regional popularity, and stormed onto the national scene during the health craze of the 1980s. Remember when TCBY first opened in your town?

Just like with mass-produced yogurt, most frozen yogurt is far from a WAMP product. Almost all frozen yogurts are loaded with processed ingredients, made of factory-farmed and processed dairy, and contain bushels of processed sugar.

The health benefits frozen yogurt claims to offer in the form of probiotics are subpar in comparison with what you'd get from eating WAMP yogurt or other WAMP fermented foods, like kimchi or miso. And any benefit you may gain may end up being negated by all the processed ingredients you need to ingest in order to consumer the good stuff in the first place.

tzatziki, a staple of Greek cuisine usually made with garlic, mint, and cucumbers, to enhance pita dishes and gyros, to cold yogurt soups called *tarator*, which are made with yogurt, cucumber, and dill—a recipe native to the Balkans.

This is the *right* way to eat yogurt. No sugar here. No fruity jams. No candy sprinkles. No toffee or apple-tart flavorings. Yogurt's natural richness comes to life when paired with ingredients that accentuate its tangy notes instead of drowning them out.

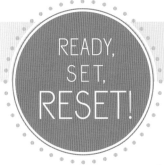

Now that you've overhauled your understanding of yogurt, it's time to overhaul the way you experience it. We will take the next three days to taste WAMP yogurt in all its flavorful glory. We will prepare it differently and savor it anew.

Plain yogurt, if made the traditional way from high-quality milk (pasture-raised and/ or organic), should taste luscious. Some of the best plain yogurt I've had in my life came from right here in the San Francisco Bay Area. A few years ago, I discovered a decadent plain yogurt from a small company called Saint Benoît Creamery in Sonoma County that produces organic, cream-top, French-style yogurt handcrafted in small batches. I spoke with the owner, Benoît Korsak, who told me he missed this traditionally made style of yogurt when he came to the United States, so he decided to make his own, using the same techniques his ancestors did back in France. His plain yogurt product is out-of-this-world delicious.

But wait. Are you still thinking that you'll miss your fruity yogurts? No problem! Fruit-flavored yogurt—if made in a WAMP way—can blow your taste buds away. I've included some recipes below as substitutes for the processed fruit-flavored yogurts you find in supermarkets. After you taste these, you'll have a hard time going back. Because these recipes call for fresh whole fruit, honey, and lemon zest—all WAMP ingredients with powerful flavors—they're designed to electrify your palate.

Instructions

Your three days will work like this. You'll omit all processed yogurts from your life for seventy-two hours. During that time, you will eat only WAMP yogurt, using the recipes below. You don't have to make all three recipes over the three days, but if you do, you'll experience broader flavors and end up enjoying yogurt on a deeper level. If you'd like to stick to just one recipe, though, that's OK too.

These recipes are very simple to make. They may require more work than going to the grocery store and buying processed yogurt, sure, but the additional effort is minimal and all recipes can me made in less than fifteen minutes. Easy!

TIPS & TOOLS for EACH DAY

Day One

Today you'll begin your path to restoring your cravings for WAMP yogurt for good. Congratulations!

If you usually start your day with a processed yogurt (any yogurt or yogurt drink that's not plain), this is your opportunity to swap it with the recipes below. For breakfast, you'll probably want to use the first recipe—it's very quick. If you don't have fresh raspberries or apricots, go with anything in your kitchen that's ripe: peaches, strawberries, blueberries, or bananas. Any ripe, whole fruit will do. Just give it a mash and add.

If you usually enjoy yogurt for lunch, this recipe isn't hard to accomplish at work. You can bring along a cup of plain yogurt and simply mash some fruit in a paper cup with the back of a plastic fork. There are many ways to improvise! Alternatively, you can opt not to do much until the evening, when you have more time and can explore WAMP yogurt at home in a more relaxed fashion.

In any case, on this first day, notice yogurt around you. See what kinds of yogurt they sell at your local supermarket or office pantry. What are the ingredients? How many times do you see "sugar" on the ingredient list, and in what forms (dextrose, evaporated cane sugar, corn syrup, etc.)? How many ingredients are listed overall?

Day Two

Today you're likely on a roll if you've already tried a recipe yesterday. You've probably now realized how much more delectable whole and minimally processed yogurt dishes are compared to store-bought plastic cups of the stuff.

As you did yesterday, be on the lookout today for yogurt that surrounds you. Ask your friends and family what they know about the yogurt they're eating. Do they think it's healthy? Do they know how much sugar is in it? Do they know that yogurt, on its own, should taste deliciously sour, not sweet? Do they know a lot of flavored yogurts are made using lab-created "natural flavorings"? See what they say. It will be interesting to hear these responses.

Tonight, try making the Raita recipe if you haven't done so already. Notice how it tastes. Let your taste buds experience the flavor of sour matched with spicy and the pungency that comes with raw onions. For some people, it may take some getting used to at first, but for many, yogurt this way is just as delicious as yogurt spiked with sweetness.

Day Three

Today's your last Reset day. If you have some extra time today, make your way to the supermarket if you haven't already done so to check out the yogurt aisle. Most grocery stores carry so much processed yogurt, it's mind-boggling. Take a look at just how many yogurt flavors there are, and how sugar is in everything—*particularly the yogurt that's aimed at children.* You'll realize that even yogurts boasting they're healthier than the others are processed products. See how many times "natural" and "artificial" flavorings turn up on ingredient lists. Look for stabilizers and thickeners.

Take this last day to deeply experience sourness. Before making your last recipe, take a taste of just the yogurt itself, plain. Can you taste that tanginess? That's what yogurt is all about—that bold and unique flavor—a flavor we can't pick up from any other food. It's a sourness that should be celebrated!

Enjoy the tzatziki recipe today and think about how easy it is to re-create these dishes on your own. After the Reset, you can return to these recipes and tailor them to your newly sharpened taste buds' preferences. Enjoy the versatility, and enjoy your new love of WAMP yogurt!

After the Reset

After doing this Reset, you should have a completely new relationship with yogurt. The experience alone is a grand lesson—one that you'll likely never forget. Consider it a three-day seminar where you've been present, and you've taken the time to reflect on yogurt. You now have the knowledge and tools to find WAMP yogurt, and you now realize how most yogurt, even though it's marketed as a health food, is not.

You now also have a new understanding of the taste of sour—the taste of true, pure, WAMP yogurt. Knowing this, in and of itself, is a huge win for many of us!

YOUR YOGURT RESET GROCERY LIST

- [ ] 32 oz tub plain yogurt (full or low-fat from pasture-fed cows or sheep, if possible)
- [ ] Whole cumin seeds or ground cumin
- [ ] Chili powder
- [ ] 1 red onion
- [ ] A few ripe heirloom or roma tomatoes or 1/2 cup of cherry tomatoes
- [ ] Cilantro
- [ ] Sea salt
- [ ] 1 c (8oz) Greek yogurt (organic or grass-fed)
- [ ] 1 bulb garlic
- [ ] 1 English cucumber
- [ ] 1 bunch mint
- [ ] 1 bunch dill
- [ ] 1 lemon
- [ ] Ground paprika
- [ ] Extra-virgin olive oil
- [ ] Pitted olives
- [ ] 1 package 100% whole-wheat pita bread
- [ ] Organic honey (preferably raw)
- [ ] 2 small ripe apricots or nectarines, other ripe stone fruit, or ripe pear
- [ ] 1 package ripe raspberries

By completing this Reset you now have the culinary knowledge to enjoy WAMP yogurt in a variety of fun and simple ways. You can make spicy and savory yogurt side dishes to complement proteins or other main courses. You can also whip up sweetened yogurt for your kids without having to turn to sugar-laden, store-bought yogurt. You're empowered.

Of course, you don't have to eat yogurt this way forever. Life is busy, and sometimes we need to reach for the convenient, brand-name, six-ounce plastic cups of yogurt. And that's OK. But for many of you, after tasting how delicious WAMP yogurt can be, I'm certain you'll be making some permanent changes to your yogurt consumption in the years to come. Enjoy!

Roasted Cumin and Tomato Raita

Raita is a staple yogurt-based dish of Indian cuisine, used as a condiment, relish, or side dish eaten with main courses like chicken curries and biryani's. This raita is a wonderful introduction to eating yogurt in a savory and spicy way as opposed to the sweet way in which we have been conditioned to eat it in America. When savory and spicy ingredients combine with yogurt's creamy sourness, a brilliant flavor comes to life! Raita can be prepared in many forms using ingredients like cucumbers, papayas, mangos, radishes, and even bananas and pomegranate arils. The version here is meant to be basic and requires ingredients you likely already have in your kitchen.

SERVES: 2–4
TOTAL TIME: 10 MINUTES

INGREDIENTS

- 1 c plain yogurt
- 2 tsp whole cumin seeds (use 3/4 to 1 teaspoon ground)
- 1/4 to 1/2 tsp chili powder
- 1/2 plus 1/8 c thinly sliced red onion (sliced from root to stem)
- 1/2 c ripe heirloom, Roma, or cherry tomatoes, small dice or thinly sliced
- Leaves from 8 sprigs fresh cilantro plus extra for garnish
- 1/8 tsp sea salt (optional)

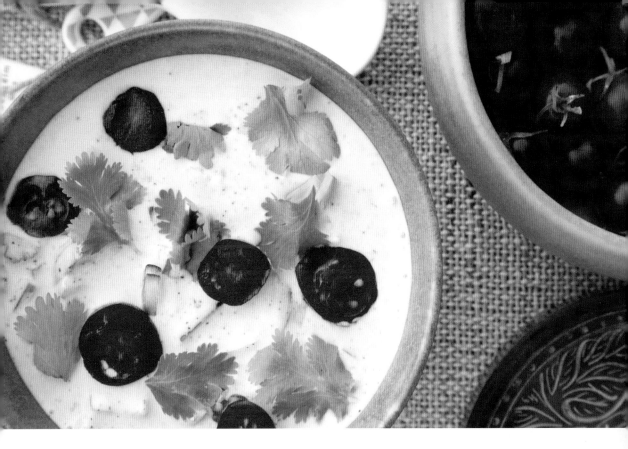

PROCEDURE

1. Set a saucepan over medium-high heat. Add cumin seeds and pan roast for a minute or so. Remove from heat and allow to cool for another minute. Transfer seeds to a spice or coffee grinder and grind, or grind using a mortar and pestle. At this point you will have extra ground cumin, as you only need 3/4 to 1 teaspoon for this recipe. (You may store the remaining if you wish or use for making the recipe again).

2. Place all ingredients in serving bowl and stir to fully incorporate. Garnish with more cilantro. Plate and serve!

Note: The keys to this recipe are proportion and fresh ground cumin. The right amount of spiciness from onions and spices offsets the cooling properties of the yogurt and the sweetness of tomatoes. Tasting as you go is key. Although you may use ground cumin from your spice rack, this recipe tests legions better using fresh ground cumin seeds—the aroma is magical!

Easy Tzatziki

YOGURT RESET RECIPE

Tzatziki, a cold Greek dish, is a recipe you can whip up in minutes in your kitchen, perfect as an appetizer for gatherings with friends or as a side dish. Think of it as the European version of raita. In fact, its name is derived from the Turkish word for chutney: *cacik*. As with raita, there are a few variations of tzatziki, but in it's most basic form, it consists of yogurt, cucumbers, dill, lemon juice, and olive oil. It tastes best as an appetizer when combined with warm toasted pita and olives.

SERVES: 4
TOTAL TIME: 5 MINUTES

INGREDIENTS

- 1 c Greek yogurt
- 1/8 to 1/4 tsp sea salt
- 2 small garlic cloves, peeled and very finely minced
- 6-inch piece English cucumber or any thin cucumber, peeled, and small dice
- 10 fresh mint leaves, finely chopped
- Fresh dill from 3 to 4 sprigs, finely chopped
- 1 tbsp lemon juice
- Ground paprika, to taste
- 1–2 tsp extra virgin olive oil

ACCOMPANIMENTS

- Olives
- Whole wheat pita bread, toasted and cut into triangles

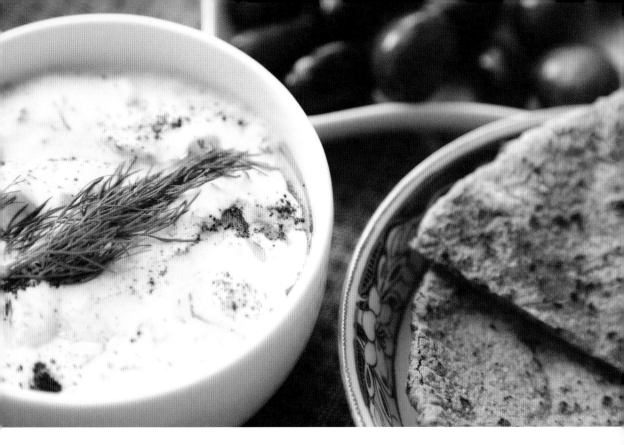

PROCEDURE

1. Place yogurt in a serving bowl, then add salt, garlic and cucumbers. Stir to combine.

2. Add remaining ingredients except olive oil and paprika, stirring again. Then drizzle olive oil over the top and garnish with a few pinches of paprika, to taste.

Note: Traditionally, tzatziki is made using strained (Greek-style) yogurt from sheep or goats milk. In this recipe, I am using Greek yogurt from cow's milk, as it's the most accessible. For more super-charged flavor, dress pita bread with olive oil, and sprinkle za'atar—a spice blend of herbs, sesame and salt—over the top. Bake until crispy. Allow to cool before cutting into triangles.

Perfectly Sweet Yogurt Three Ways

Yogurt is healthiest and most delicious when its natural sour flavor is complemented by subtle WAMP sweetness, not harsh processed sugars. These three incredibly simple recipes will eclipse any fruit-on-the-bottom, fruit blended, or honey-infused packaged yogurt cup you buy from the grocery store because the ingredients you are using are fresh and whole. The flavor is unmatched. You'll find it hard to go back to peel back cups again!

SERVES: 1 PER CUP
TOTAL TIME: 5 MINUTES

INGREDIENTS (INCLUDES ALL THREE RECIPES)

- 6 oz plain yogurt for each variation (full or low-fat from pasture-fed cows or sheep if possible)
- 1/2 tsp (or slightly more, to taste) USDA organic honey or raw honey
- Zest of 1/4 small lemon
- 2 small apricots, seed removed, muddled or blended in small food processor
- 1/4 c organic or farmers market fresh raspberries, crushed

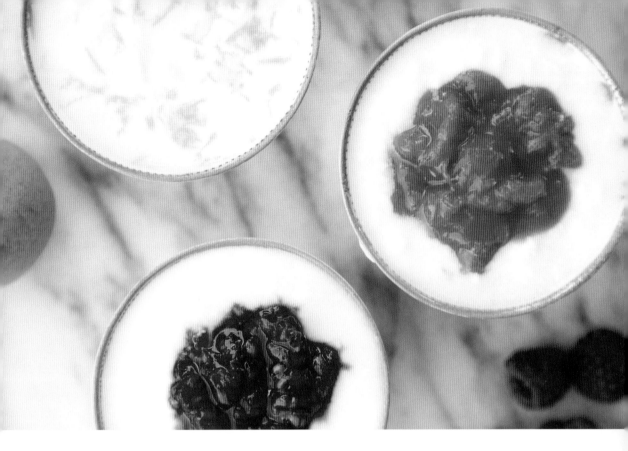

PROCEDURES:

Perfectly Sweet Yogurt with Honey

Place yogurt in a cup, drizzling honey on top, stir to incorporate. Zest the lemon and transfer zest to the cup. Stir again to fully incorporate. Enjoy!

Perfectly Sweet Yogurt with Apricots

Place yogurt in a cup. Spoon apricots on top.

Note: If apricots are very ripe and soft, using the back of a fork is enough to crush fruit in the bottom of a bowl. Otherwise, using a small blender is a good option.

Perfectly Sweet Yogurt with Raspberries

Place yogurt in a cup. Spoon raspberries on top. Stir to fully incorporate.

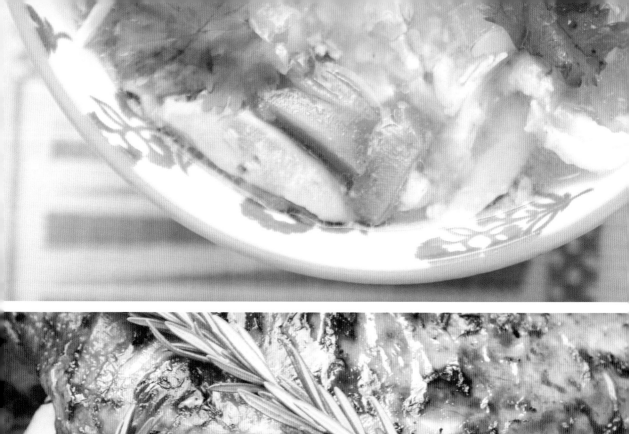

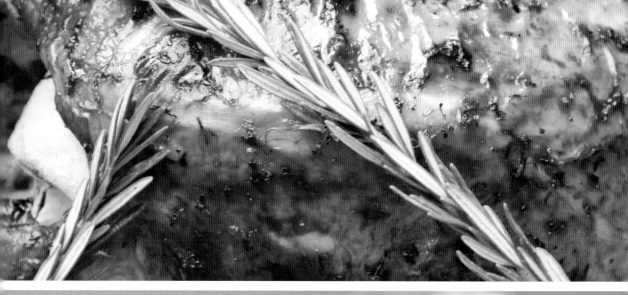

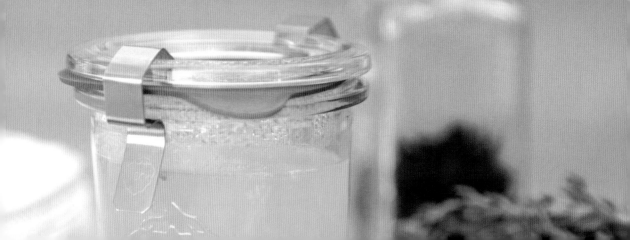

Chicken
RESET

When it comes to chicken, most of us (who aren't vegetarians) eat it mindlessly and often. Consuming so much chicken seems de rigueur. It shows up on menus as if it's expected to be there, and we never question it. In fact, chicken has snuck its way into just about every meal of our day, from chicken sausages for breakfast to grilled chicken sandwiches for lunch and General Tso's chicken for dinner. But there's too much we don't know about what we're putting in our bodies.

It seems as though we can get chicken—known scientifically as the *Gallus gallus domesticus*—any way we want it. There's chicken lunchmeat, chicken tenders, chicken breasts, chicken fingers, chicken wings, shredded chicken, boneless chicken, diced chicken, fried chicken, barbecued chicken, and let's not forget chicken nuggets, my hands-down childhood favorite. "Dad, can we get another order of the six-piece McNuggets, *please?*"

Perhaps chicken is everywhere because it's become the answer to our nation's obsession with protein that can be easily packaged for our on-the-go lifestyle. There's no need for plates, forks, or even tables when you can eat chicken fingers in the car or chicken-salad sandwiches standing up. Chicken has become our nation's premier convenience protein.

Yet, regardless of why we eat so much of it, we're eating it all *wrong*. The kind of chicken we're eating these days is not as healthy as it can be, and it misses the mark when it comes to flavor. The truth of the matter, sad as it may be, is that the majority of us have only experienced mediocre chicken flavor *over the course of our entire lives*.

Just about a half century ago, our relationship with chicken was much more real, more WAMP. In 1962, we bought 83 percent of our chicken in whole form, butchering a bird into its requisite parts in the comfort of our own kitchens. Today, we buy only about 11 percent of chicken in its whole form. What this means is that not only have we lost touch with chicken and the animal it comes from, but we've also lost our ancestors' skills for enjoying it in the right way.

All those precut, cellophane-wrapped parts from Tyson do us no favors. For example, thanks to our obsession with "lean protein," we prefer chicken breasts (which now account for nearly 60 percent of chicken-part purchases) to drumsticks, yet breasts are the most taste-deficient cut of all, and also the hardest to cook well. Our preference for skinless and boneless doesn't help either, as both are required for big-time chicken flavor, succulence, and aroma as well as vital nutrients. Cooking with chicken bones, especially in stocks and soups, is an age-old tradition that yields dishes high in calcium and other nutrients. Sure, you reduce fat when you cook without them, but you miss out on all their health-boosting properties. Isn't that what chicken soup is for?

The transgressions with poultry don't stop there. With 95 percent of chicken now coming from factory-farming operations, we're no longer eating pure chicken. Eating factory-farmed chicken is just one more way we're losing out on nourishment and flavor.

And, with about 48 percent of chicken sold to us as processed products, we've lost our way when it comes to eating WAMP. Everything from frozen patties and lunchmeats to strips and buffalo wings requires countless feats of food processing. And processing, as we know, means a high dependency on refined salt, sugar, wheat, and fat and a host of lab-concocted additives. McDonald's McNuggets aren't just breast meat that's battered and fried; they're filled with leavening agents (e.g., aluminum phosphate), processed sugars, flavorings, refined flours, and other synthetic ingredients. In other words, you can't make chicken nuggets or the frozen patties you buy at the grocery store in your own kitchen from scratch—they're not WAMP foods.

Our relationship with chicken needs a serious reset. It's time to take pause, reflect, and completely overhaul our connection with the *Gallus gallus domesticus*, rebooting the way we know it, buy it, cook it, and crave it.

> In 1962, we bought 83 percent of our chicken in whole form, butchering a bird into its requisite parts in the comfort of our own kitchens. Today, we buy only about 11 percent of chicken in its whole form.

The Egg Came First: What You Need to Know About Chicken

It was a shock to me to learn that chickens weren't really a significant part of the American diet until around our parents' generation. For some seven thousand years, chickens were mainly used for cockfighting, egg-laying, and even soothsaying—*not* for meals. The ancient Romans took chickens with them during wartime to foretell battles—a bird's good appetite meant a victory was at hand.

Eating chicken wasn't commonplace, as it is now. Even up until the early 1900s, chickens were mainly raised in backyards, providing their owners with a steady source of eggs. Only when the hens became too old to lay would there be a roast chicken for Sunday night dinner. In other words, poultry was considered a "special occasion" food, something households had but once in a while. If you didn't own a chicken, you'd have to be lucky enough to buy one from a nice neighbor who was willing to sell.

Chickens raised specifically for their meat, in a commercial fashion, became known as "broilers" by the 1920s, yet still played second fiddle to the commercial egg industry. It wouldn't be until 1952 that commercial broilers overtook backyard farm chickens as the most popular poultry, thanks in part to the rationing of beef, pork, and veal during World War II. Then, roughly two decades later, commercial chicken morphed into an integrated mega-industry positioned mainly in the deep rural South—an area dubbed the "Broiler Belt"—where technological innovations and scientific manipulation of feed made it possible to produce poultry in vast quantities year round. This marked the beginning of what we now consider poultry factory-farming operations—a highly concentrated industry composed of only a handful of players, including Tyson Foods and Perdue Farms.

By the late 1970s, chicken went through yet another evolution, this time thanks to the golden arches. According to Eric Schlosser, author of *Fast Food Nation*, in 1979, McDonald's chairman, Fred Turner, asked his suppliers to come up with a boneless chicken menu offering about the "size of his thumb" that wouldn't compete with the chain's mainline product, the hamburger. At this time in our country, new medical research was touting the benefits of lowering saturated fat and cholesterol consumption, and red meats. Steaks and hamburgers, suddenly became out of fashion in favor of leaner protein like chicken breast. Turner wanted to capitalize on this sea change in consumer demand. Six months later, the "McNugget" was born, made of "reconstituted chicken, composed mainly of breast meat, that was held together by stabilizers, breaded, fried, frozen, then reheated"—all procedures that required the best that food science and food processing had to offer.

This bite-sized invention, officially launched in 1983, changed America's relationship with chicken overnight. Now challenged to meet cravings for the McNugget, McDonald's became the nation's second largest buyer of chicken (Kentucky Fried Chicken was the first), and Tyson Foods, one of its suppliers, even created *a whole new breed of bird,* one with larger breasts, just to keep up with McNugget-fueled demand.

With chicken officially on the map, made in mass and consumed in quantity, convenience became king. Instead of consuming chicken whole, as we had for millennia, we started eating chicken almost exclusively in processed and precut forms: as butchered parts, as eat-while-you-drive fast-food creations, and in the form of chicken hot dogs, chicken lunchmeat, and chicken bologna. All three of the latter are products created using "mechanically separated chicken" (MSC), a paste-like product made by forcing chicken parts through a sieve-like device under high pressure to separate meat from the bone, a food-processing method used in the industry since the 1960s.

By 2010, poultry had outrun beef as the most popular meat in the nation, and to this day it still holds the number-one slot. Americans eat more chicken now than anyone else on planet Earth—approximately 83 pounds per person each year.

Incredibly, over a span of just fifty years, the domesticated chicken went from being viewed as a prized indulgence at a Sunday dinner to a run-of-the-mill offering at our local Olive Garden.

> Factory-farmed chicken is nothing more than "filler food."

Super WAMP Chicken Tastes Like Chicken!

These days, 95 percent of chickens we consume in America aren't happy. And the reason is simple: They're not healthy. Why does their health matter to us? Because healthier chicken makes for tastier chicken.

Factory-bred chickens don't live the way they're meant to. Remember the Super WAMP category of foods from page 26? Factory-farmed chickens can't be classified as such because the way they're farmed is not in concert with their biological requirements or the sustainability of the ecosystem.

Chickens are natural athletes. They're supposed to chase after worms and insects, to exercise their legs and bodies running outdoors, and to browse about scratching for small seeds, grasses, and leaves. Broiler chickens that come from factories, however, don't move this way. They live packed like sardines inside rearing houses: insulated, window-less warehouses about as long as a football field, where their food, drink, and light are all controlled by humans.

Because they've been specially bred in an effort to produce massive, cheap amounts of poultry product to meet our insatiable demand for wings, tenders, and grilled chicken sandwiches, these chickens have been raised to be bigger—way bigger—than their ances-tors. Factory chickens develop so rapidly that if we humans grew as fast, we'd be 349 pounds by our second birthday! Broilers get this way because they've been both selectively bred to be gigantic and fed a diet of soy meal, corn, growth-promoting antibiotics, and animals by-products—a diet that isn't in tune with their biology. And so what if they're unnaturally big? Well, the problem is that they're so fat they have trouble moving. It's been reported these birds are so huge that their bodies can't function. They couldn't even make it to a worm if they saw one. Today's chickens are eating bad food, not exercising, and needlessly drugged.

Processed Chicken:
Stouffer's Chicken Alfredo Frozen Dinner

Ingredients: Milk skim, macaroni blanched product (semolina, water, egg[s] whites), chicken meat white cooked (chicken meat white, water, tapioca starch modified, flavor[s] chicken (chicken broth dehydrated, chicken powder, **flavor[s] natural**), carrageenan, whey protein concentrate, vegetable(s) oil, corn syrup solids, sodium phosphate, salt), water, soybean oil, margarine (corn oil liquid, corn oil partially hydrogenated, milk skim, salt, **flavor[s] natural**, soy lecithin, vegetable[s] mono and diglycerides, annatto added for color, flavor(s) cheese, citric acid added to improve stability), milk cultured, milk solids non-fat cultured, datem, garlic dehydrated, cheese parmesan enzyme modified (milk cultured, water, salt, enzyme[s]), enzyme(s), **flavor(s)**, cheese granular, lactic acid, cheese mozzarella, cheese parmesan (milk cultured, salt, enzyme[s], salt, sodium citrate, spice[s], vitamin A palmitate), sour cream mix dehydrated, cheese parmesan paste, corn starch modified.

The result is nutrient-depleted and flavorless chicken. Just ask any farmer who raises chickens the right way, the way Mother Nature intended: on pasture, where they're allowed to live twice as long as factory-farmed chickens. They'll tell you that when chickens are raised on their natural diets, they have more nutrients, like conjugated linoleic acid (CLAs), a type of fat that helps combat disease. They'll tell you that when chickens are grown too fast and don't get enough sunlight or a varied diet (not just corn and soy), what we're left with is chicken that's robbed of taste—insipid and terribly bland.

Most of the chicken and chicken dishes we're buying today at the grocery store and at restaurants have compromised flavor. That's why chicken drumsticks, breasts, and thighs end up on the grill slathered with what seems like vats of Lawry's Marinade and BBQ sauce. Bland chicken is part of the reason why chicken wades in pools of butter and dipping sauces and why chicken is packed with beans and salsa in your favorite burrito: because without these flavorful accompaniments, we probably wouldn't enjoy eating it. When you strip factory chicken down to its core, it doesn't taste like much of anything. Factory-farmed chicken is nothing more than what I call a "filler food."

When it comes to processed chicken, the story gets even muddier. Processed chicken products, such as frozen breaded breast chunks, usually get their flavor from refined flours, salt, fats, sugars, and additives. In fact, flavorists—the scientists who create fragrances and flavors for companies like Nestlé and Pepsi Cola—have devised fake chicken flavoring (powders and liquids made from chemically decomposing soybeans and other substances) to mimics real chicken flavor. These additives—you'll see them on ingredient lists as "natural flavoring" or "artificial flavoring," as in the example on page 172—are often injected into frozen chicken parmesan dinners and other chicken products to make them taste "chicken-y," when in reality, they don't.

The chicken that our grandparents' generation was used to eating had a flavor profile that few of us get to experience today. Ask any chef who takes quality seriously when putting chicken on her menu and she'll tell you that the bones of pasture-raised chickens—chickens that are allowed their natural diet and exercise regimes—are stronger and more flavorful. She'll tell you that the meat is more succulent, rich, and even nutty, with more character. She'll tell you the difference in taste is unmatched.

Alas, getting our hands on WAMP chicken isn't an easy task when so many of our chickens in America are factory-bred. We must motivate ourselves to seek it out, either at a local farmers' market, a CSA, or even via phone if we live in a climate that's too cold for year-round chicken farming. This kind of chicken is indeed more costly, but it's well worth the extra effort and investment. If finding pasture-raised chicken is difficult, the next best option is "USDA organic." (See the sidebar on page 175 for more about Super WAMP chicken.)

Using the Whole Bird: A Return to Flavor

Imagine: Only fifty years ago, most American families were cooking whole chickens. Today, not only are we outsourcing half our chicken meals to restaurant chefs (57 percent of these at fast-food restaurants), but when we do end up cooking at home, we're mainly using white breast meat, the least flavorful cut.

Back in the 1960s, my father used to buy a whole bird at the grocery store. He'd come home and butcher it himself into breast, thighs, drumsticks and wings and remove the skin if a recipe called for it. Today, we think skinless, boneless chicken breast *is*

> For most of our history, making chicken has been an intricate part of family affairs, Sunday dinners, and special occasions. Chicken has, until modern times, been synonymous with heritage, hearth, and home. Time-honored family chicken dishes, like casseroles and holiday roasts, have been passed down through generations. Abraham Lincoln's favorite dish was reputedly home-cooked chicken fricassee.

chicken. The only time we might see a whole chicken is when we're reading a children's bedtime story that features barnyard animals or during a trip to a local petting zoo. With nearly all chicken precut into legs and thighs, skinned and sliced, or processed into perfectly formed patties or strips, we've stopped connecting the dots between food and fowl. We see breasts, but we don't envision the bird. We buy a boneless thigh, but we don't know where on the animal it came from. We use chicken stock, but we don't know how it got in the can or box.

Lucky for us, we can reverse course altogether by doing one thing: cooking a whole chicken. Dealing with a whole bird as opposed to its parts is a very intimate, visceral, and humbling experience. Disjointing a whole chicken, although seemingly taxing and complex, was to our grandparents' generation a necessary life skill, and one that didn't take more than a few minutes.

Working with a whole bird as opposed to just parts means legions more flavor. That's because great taste mainly resides in the parts of the chicken we usually never see—the skin, bones, and tendons. Authentic chicken flavor requires synergy amongst a variety of chicken components. Skins-on and bones-in help keep the meat moist, tender, and tasty. That's why some of the most time-honored, traditional chicken recipes, such as coq a vin, chicken casserole, and roast chicken, require using the whole chicken. This way, the bones stay in, the skin stays on, and the flavor blows our taste buds through the roof.

Super WAMP Chicken

Although skinless, boneless chicken thighs and other packaged chicken parts at the grocery store are minimally processed foods and therefore WAMP foods, I consider the parts that are the least prepped to be the best options. Try buying a whole chicken or pieces with bones still in them. And if they are from pasture-raised or organic chicken, then they're "Super WAMP," your very best choice for healthier, tastier chicken.

Working with the darker cuts of chicken, such as the legs, can also release exquisite flavor, because these darker parts are from the active areas of the chicken's body comprised of connective tissues, tendons, and ligaments. Those tendons and ligaments are made of collagen, which transforms into gelatin when cooked, releasing gorgeous juices and huge, old-fashioned flavor.

Nutrients are spread throughout various parts of a chicken. While chicken breasts are indeed nourishing, dark meat contains more iron, zinc, and various additional nutrients. By eating exclusively breast meat, we rob ourselves of the full spectrum of vitamins and minerals that chicken has to offer.

Cooking chicken in these ways can be hugely rewarding, and nothing short of a grand, multisensory experience. Imagine walking into your kitchen, the air filled with the warm, comforting aromas of chicken slowly cooking in wine and fragrant herbs like tarragon and parsley, chicken you cleaned, seasoned, and disjointed yourself.

And not only is it rewarding, delectable, and empowering to cook recipes based on an entire chicken, it's economical and just makes sense. Leftovers go in a lunch bag, neck and back go into a stock, and the need to survive solely on pricey, unsatisfying breasts vanishes.

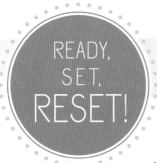

READY,
SET,
RESET!

Now that we've been educated about chicken—its history, how much of it has gone from WAMP to processed, and how much we are missing out in terms of flavor—it's time for a chicken reboot. It's time for us to reconnect with chicken on a new level, and we need to taste, touch, see, and smell chicken anew!

Instructions

Here's what you'll do. First, choose a date on your calendar when you'll have the time to dedicate to making the recipes in this Reset—they are longer than others in this book. But remember, this Reset lasts only three days, and you only have to make these three recipes once! On Day One, you'll roast a whole bird. On Day Two, you'll make a stock from scratch. And on Day Three, you'll make a delicious and fragrant chicken soup.

First thing's first. You'll need to source the chicken, which should be from a pasture-raised poultry producer if at all possible. You might want to carve out an hour or so to research places where you can find this kind of chicken in your community. Check your local farmers' market, butcher shops, CSA (community supported agriculture), or online. Look for chicken that is "pasture-raised" or "100 percent pasture-raised." Note that these chickens don't have to be labeled "USDA Organic."

If you can't find a pasture-raised chicken, the next best option is a "USDA Organic" chicken. Poultry labeled "USDA Organic" must have access to the outdoors and cannot be given antibiotics or growth hormones, and must be fed an organic diet (it may be a diet of organic corn and soy). Generally speaking, you'll want to find chickens that have been raised in a way that closely resembles the way they should live in nature.

Be careful when reading labels! Currently, hormones are not allowed in poultry in accordance with USDA standards. That's good. But if the chicken is labeled "free range" or "free roaming," this doesn't guarantee that the bird even set one foot outdoors over the course of its life; it only means that poultry producers demonstrated to the USDA that the poultry was allowed *access* to the outside.

"Natural" is another term that tends to be misleading. Although the USDA recognizes and regulates this term for poultry, it does not refer to how the chickens were raised, but *only how they were processed*. "Natural" poultry must be free of artificial colors, flavors, sweeteners, preservatives, and other such ingredients when it is processed into its final product. Therefore, for this Reset, steer clear of this label. Instead, go for pasture-raised or USDA Organic, and don't be afraid to ask, ask, ask! When you're at the meat counter, query the butcher about where the chicken you're buying came from, and whether he knows any other details he can share with you. Be curious.

Be prepared to pony up more cash in purchasing your chicken over these three days. It's a short period to experience the best chicken has to offer. The sacrifice will be well worth the investment.

Last, throughout the course of this Reset, you will abstain from any other chicken dishes you don't cook yourself, particularly processed and prepared chicken meals. By doing so, you'll be making an effort to think more about the provenance, quantity, and quality of chicken you've been eating in your everyday life.

TIPS & TOOLS for EACH DAY

Day One—Roast Chicken

Welcome to the first day of your Chicken Reset! If you've never had the chance to roast a whole chicken in your kitchen, today may change your life. And even if you have, you may still be in for a great experience. If you're home today, you may want to think of making this recipe for lunch or dinner; it will take a little under an hour.

What you'll realize right off the bat is that this recipe is comically simple. After you place the bird in your oven, there's no need to babysit it. Go off and do something else in the meantime. As the bird is roasting, you'll notice that your kitchen (and your

First thing's first. You'll need to source the chicken, which should be from a pasture-raised poultry producer if at all possible. Check your local farmer's market, butcher shops, CSA, or online.

home) will start to smell divine. Take time to savor the aroma and enjoy the satisfaction that comes along with it!

When your roast is ready, you may want to have warm rice, or a salad alongside (see recipes in the Salad Reset, or Tabouli from the Wheat Reset). Indulge in the satisfaction of pulling it out of the oven, letting it sit, and carving it yourself. Have the first bite and notice the juiciness, tenderness, and crispness all at once. You'll realize that there are few better ways to experience chicken in the world.

In general, enjoy the fruits of your labor and make sure you tell your friends what you've done. Ask them when was the last time they roasted a whole chicken. Tell them how easy and rewarding and delicious it was. Compare it with buying rotisserie chicken at the store.

And share your recipe! When I gave this recipe to my neighbors recently, the next time they came over to the house, they said they'd already made it three times and joked about how they wanted to start a roast chicken business!

Day Two—Chicken Stock

Today will be another eye-opening experience for those who haven't had the opportunity to make a stock from scratch. Making a stock (or broth) dates back to ancient times. Stock is considered the foundation of great cooking. Cultures all over the world have been making stocks to nourish themselves for centuries. The French, Italians, Chinese, Japanese, Africans, South Americans, and Russians use stock as the basis of their traditional cuisines. Stock is used as a base to add flavor in countless recipes from soups to gravies. Famous French chef and culinary writer Auguste Escoffier proclaimed, "Indeed, stock is everything in cooking. Without it, nothing can be done." A flavorful stock is key to making stews taste delectable and sauces rich and satisfying.

From a health perspective, stocks have been used as a healing food for generations. When bones, cartilage, and tendons are simmered in liquid for long periods of time, they

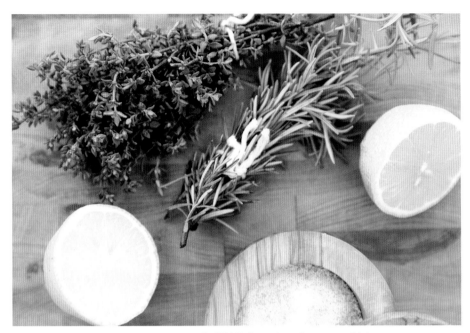

Herbs, lemon zest, and sea salt—simple WAMP flavorings for roast chicken

impart a bevy of key nutrients that can easily be absorbed by our bodies, such as calcium, magnesium, phosphorus, silicon, sulfur, and trace minerals. Making homemade stock is an age-old tradition that's been lost with the creation of bouillon cubes and canned and boxed premade stock and broth. The problem with those? They're not fresh, they're processed, and they're not as yummy.

When you're making this stock, think about how infrequently we use chicken parts—for example, the back and the neck—and how much of a whole chicken usually goes to waste when all we're after at the grocery store is boneless breast meat.

Making stock from scratch is a beautiful and empowering experience. If you thought making a roast was easy, this is even easier. After you put all your ingredients into your pot, you're hands-free. Leave the kitchen and tend to other things!

Just as with the roast chicken, you'll soon smell gorgeous aromas enveloping your house. Notice and enjoy them. Take pride in the fact that you now know how to replicate those tiny cubes and cans of stock that you've been using for years. Revel in the fact that you now know what goes into making many of the foods you may have once

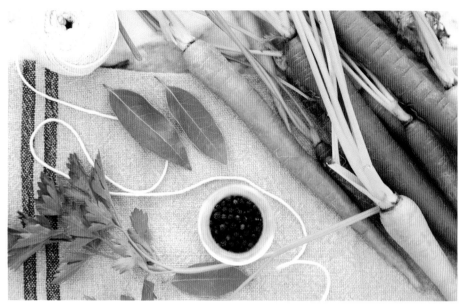

WAMP chicken stock ingredients: peppercorn, carrots, parsley, bay leaves

thought complicated and/or mysterious. Ratatouille, rice pilaf, peppercorn steak sauce and risotto are all made with stock.

When your stock is done, be sure to taste it so you can compare it with the premade, processed stocks you've bought in the past. Keep two to three cups in the fridge for your next recipe—the chicken soup.

Also, note how inexpensive it is to make stock. All you need are some vegetables and chicken parts, which tend to be relatively cheap compared to skinless, boneless breasts or thighs. From this one recipe alone, you'll be able to store several cups of stock in your freezer to use in the future.

Day Three—Classic Chicken Soup

Dubbed "Jewish penicillin," chicken soup is one of those recipes that should be in everyone's culinary arsenal. A soup that's been used as a medicinal remedy for colds and flus for centuries, chicken soup has earned a reputation as the ultimate under-the-weather food.

On this third and last day of your Reset, think about how rewarding it is to make chicken soup from scratch, not having to rely on Campbell's soup out of the can. As you cook this last recipe, savor the fact that you can now confidently nourish your family, your kids, and even yourself with an ancient and classic dish.

Remember, you don't have to take a lot of care in cutting your vegetables and prepping for this dish; chicken soup is supposed to be rustic and casual.

When your soup is done and cool enough to eat, note how different it tastes from a chicken soup you'd buy in a can, or chicken soup you've experienced at a restaurant. Check in with yourself and realize how empowering it feels to nourish yourself with a dish you've made with your own two hands.

> Check in with yourself and realize how empowering it feels to nourish yourself with a dish you've made with your own two hands.

On this last day, take a minute to talk about chicken with your friends and family. How do other people connect with chicken on a daily basis? Do they realize how many parts of a chicken they never get the chance to see or taste? Do they know just how much chicken is processed in our food supply? Have they ever roasted a whole chicken before?

Finally, note just how crucial a good, fresh stock is to a soup like this. A ton of flavor came from the stock you made yesterday!

After the Reset

Congratulations on graduating from your Chicken Reset! This Reset, like those before it, is meant to overhaul your thinking, and get you craving WAMP chicken.

You now have a greater appreciation for chicken: its history, its provenance, how it gets to your plate, and how it serves to nourish you and others. You're now aware that a lot of chicken dishes we eat aren't WAMP or Super WAMP. You now know that even though a chicken nugget is supposedly made with breast meat, it's not that simple.

Now that you know a lot more about chicken labeling and how to find the healthiest, happiest chicken, you'll start asking your butcher and servers more questions. You'll start reading labels on the frozen herb roasted chicken dinner you're thinking about buying more carefully. You now know that a lot of the flavor you once believed came from chicken really comes from "natural flavors" that have been added to it.

YOUR CHICKEN RESET GROCERY LIST

- ☐ 3–4 lb pasture-raised or USDA organic chicken
- ☐ Olive oil
- ☐ Rosemary
- ☐ 3 lemons
- ☐ Sea salt
- ☐ Ground pepper
- ☐ Thyme (optional)
- ☐ Sage (optional)
- ☐ 2 1/2–3 lbs pasture raised or organic meaty chicken parts (backs, wings, necks)

- ☐ 2 large onions
- ☐ 1 large bulb garlic
- ☐ 1 bunch carrots
- ☐ Celery
- ☐ Parsley
- ☐ Peppercorns
- ☐ Whole clove
- ☐ Bay leaves
- ☐ 2–2 1/2 lbs pasture-raised or organic whole chicken legs (about three), skin removed

Best of all, this Reset has likely made you fall in love with chicken in a deeper, more intimate way. After experiencing the aroma and warmth of homemade chicken dishes, you see just how pleasurable it is to enjoy WAMP chicken in this new way. Skinless breasts can't compare to a whole roast or a soup made with homemade stock—it's chicken on a completely different level.

Now, I'm not suggesting you shouldn't ever have a chicken sandwich from Burger King. Remember, it's all about the 80/20 Rule. If you like what you've learned and want to make WAMP chicken a bigger part of your life, just focus on eating it that way 80 percent of the time. Still, one good rule of thumb is to try to stay away from packaged and frozen, prepared chicken dishes and fast-food chicken *as much as possible.*

You can make the recipes you created during this Reset again and again, and share them with your friends and family—invite them over for a roast chicken dinner or offer your chicken soup when they're feeling under the weather!

Lemon and Rosemary Roast Chicken

This simple recipe will fast become a family favorite in your home! The use of fresh rosemary, lemons, and lemon zest impart huge flavor and aroma to this nourishing and beautiful WAMP dish.

SERVES: 4
TOTAL TIME: 1 HOUR

TOOLS

* Roasting pan, tray, or tin
* Baster (optional)
* Thermometer (optional)
* Aluminum foil

INGREDIENTS

* 3–4 lb pasture-raised chicken (USDA Organic is next best option)
* 2 tbsp olive oil
* 1 tbsp chopped rosemary
* 2 tsp lemon zest from organic lemon
* Several generous pinches sea salt
* 1/4 tsp ground pepper, or 10 turns of pepper mill
* 2 lemons, sliced in half
* 2 sprigs rosemary
* 2 sprigs thyme (optional)
* 2 sprigs sage (optional)

PROCEDURE

1. Preheat oven to 400°F, using convection setting, if possible. Thoroughly wash chicken with cold water, both outside and inside the cavity. Remove giblets (you may use all in the stock recipe tomorrow with the exception of the liver, which tends to lend a bitter taste). Pat dry. Lay chicken, breast side up, in the roasting pan.

2. In a small bowl, blend chopped rosemary with lemon zest and olive oil. Pour over chicken and spread evenly using your hands. Place herbs inside the cavity. Squeeze lemon juice over the chicken (a squeeze or two from one lemon half) and tuck all four halves inside the cavity with herbs. Season with a few generous pinches of salt and pepper.

3. You may wish to tuck the wings underneath and tie the legs together with kitchen twine to help the bird keep its shape while cooking. Place chicken in the oven and cook for about 50 minutes to 1 hour (depending on size of bird and your oven's true temperature), making sure to baste chicken with drippings/juices throughout (to keep the chicken moist and succulent). Cook until chicken's internal temperature reaches 165°F, using a meat thermometer in the thickest part of the thigh. Remove chicken from the oven and set it aside, letting it cool for 10 minutes. You may wish to tent it with aluminum foil to keep it warm. Then carve and serve it.

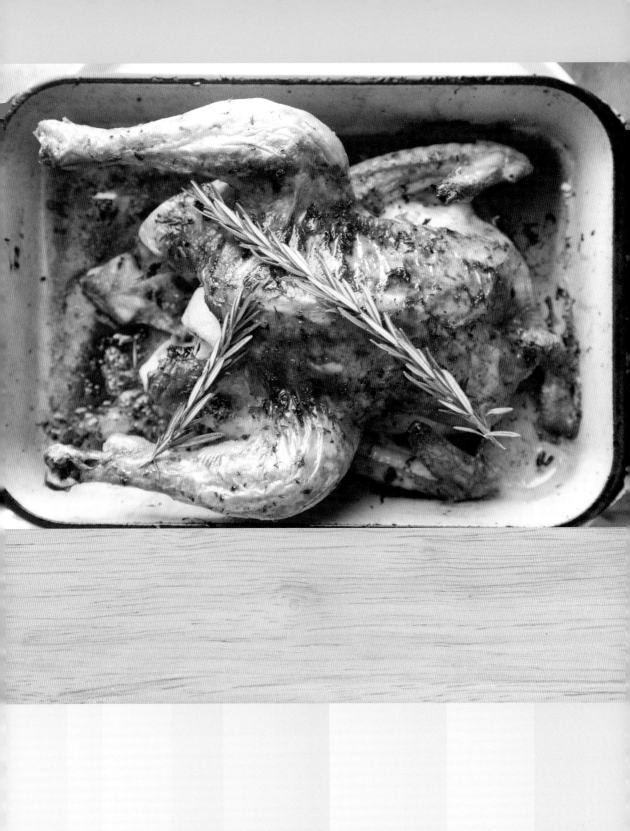

Chicken Stock

This chicken stock is simple to make and so much more nourishing than any stock or broth you'll find at the grocery store. Your kitchen will smell amazing, too!

YIELD: 16+ CUPS
TOTAL TIME: 4 HOURS

INGREDIENTS

- 2 1/2 to 3 lbs pasture-raised or organic meaty chicken parts (backs, wings, necks)
- 1 onion, peeled
- 4–5 garlic cloves, unpeeled
- 2 medium carrots, peeled
- 1 stalk celery
- 1 tsp sea salt
- 20 c cold, filtered water
- Giblets without liver (optional)

TIE IN A CHEESECLOTH (BOUQUET GARNI):

- Few sprigs parsley
- Few sprigs thyme (optional)
- 1/2 tsp peppercorns
- 1 whole clove
- 1 bay leaf

PROCEDURE

1. Place all ingredients and cheesecloth-tied bouquet garni into a deep stockpot (a 10- to 12-quart pot works best). Add water, cover, and bring almost to a boil (you don't want to bring it to full boil as fat and scum can make the stock cloudy at

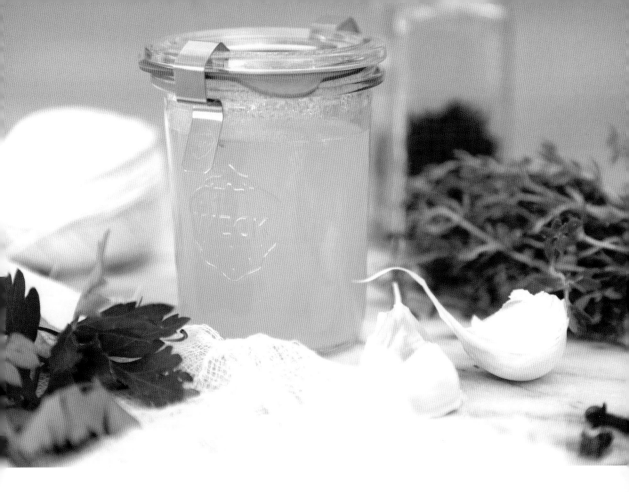

that temperature); then lower to a simmer (i.e., a gentle boil whereby small bubbles break the surface intermittently), and skim off any scum (not fat) that has reached the surface using a ladle.

2. Partially cover, leaving a small 1/2 to 1-inch opening for steam to escape. Gently simmer for about 4 hours.

3. Strain the stock through a colander or sieve, discarding the remaining vegetables and bones. If you're planning to use any for another recipe right away, skim all fat from the top using a ladle. Otherwise, allow stock to completely cool to room temperature. Then transfer it to containers and either refrigerate (for up to three or four days, skimming fat when you're ready to use it) or freeze it (up to about three months). Before you use this stock again, you'll want to heat it back to a full boil to ensure it's safe for consumption.

Chicken and Brown Rice Soup

This wildly flavorful soup will nourish your friends and family for years to come. I've used brown rice here to show off the flavor of WAMP rice versus white refined rice—it's tastier and gives this soup a fantastic texture.

SERVES: 6–8
TOTAL TIME: 1 HOUR

INGREDIENTS

- 2 tsp extra-virgin olive oil
- 4 garlic cloves, peeled and pounded once or twice
- 1 large onion, peeled and chopped
- 4 medium-sized carrots, unpeeled, scrubbed clean, coarsely chopped
- 2–3 stalks celery, roughly chopped into 1/2-inch pieces
- 1 bay leaf
- 1 tsp sea salt
- 1 c short-grain brown rice, rinsed
- 2 c chicken stock from recipe on page 186
- 6 c filtered water
- 2–2 1/2 lbs pasture-raised or organic chicken legs (thigh plus drumstick), skin removed

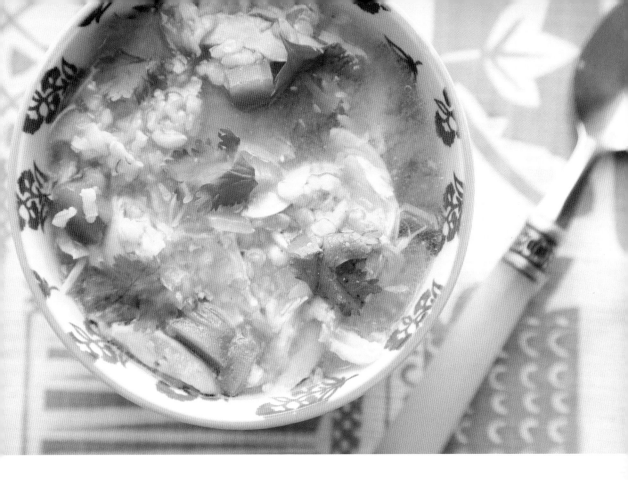

PROCEDURE

1. In Dutch oven or large heavy-bottomed soup pot, warm oil over medium heat. Add garlic and onions and stir. Cook until onions become translucent.

2. Add carrots and celery, and cook another couple of minutes. Add a bit of stock if the onions begin to brown (onions should stay translucent).

3. Add all remaining ingredients, cover, and bring to a boil. Lower to a simmer and cook, covered, for 45 minutes.

4. Remove chicken legs and shred meat off the bones using a large fork and knife. Return the meat to the pot, discarding bones.

5. Cook for another 5 minutes or until rice is completely cooked. Add more salt, if necessary. Enjoy immediately.

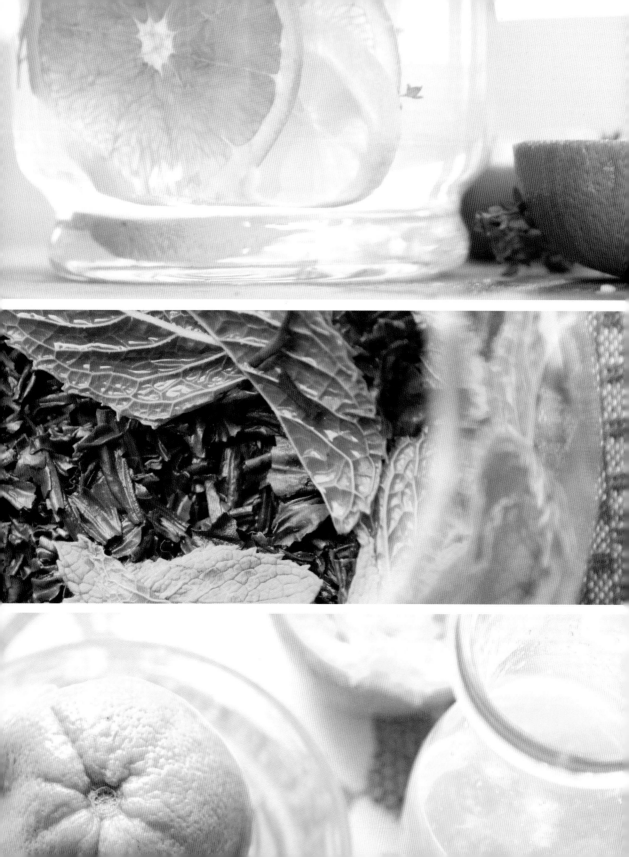

Beverage
RESET

When I was a kid, I never thought about what I was drinking. Because beverages went down so easily and quickly, I probably didn't consider them to be as important as solid food. I just had a Capri Sun or Tropicana whenever I felt thirsty. I wasn't conscious about the drinks that surrounded me, and I certainly didn't think that what I sipped had any ramifications on my health or on how much I enjoyed healthy food.

It wasn't until college that I began the switch to healthier options like water, and it wouldn't be until even later in my twenties that I started investigating the beverages at the grocery store, in restaurants, and in office vending machines. What I found would eventually and indelibly alter my relationship with drinks forever.

From bottled iced cappuccinos to energy drinks to kiwi-flavored iced teas, the beverages that flood our culture today are nothing more than processed liquids doused with processed sugars. They're not suited to our biological make-up; they're not WAMP.

For the majority of our history, the beverages we drank had few, if any, additional ingredients. Nowadays, there are dozens of funny-sounding words on ingredient lists: things like "sodium benzoate," "sucralose," "corn syrup," "evaporated cane juice," "ascorbic acid," "natural flavor," and "Yellow #5." I've even seen "canola oil" on some.

And the sugar content is off the charts. Refined and processed sweeteners dominate ingredient lists. In fact, there's so much sugar in our beverages that nearly half of the added sugar in our diet comes from drinks alone—approximately eleven teaspoons of sugar per day. We know from the Sugar Reset chapter that by playing on our innate weakness for sweet taste, processed sugars manipulate our cravings and deaden the sensitivity of our taste buds so much that we end up having a hard time reaching for healthier beverages like green tea that aren't so sugary. In other words, we end up not enjoying the beverages that love us back.

> We weren't *buying* beverages when we got thirsty. We were drawing them from wells, milking them from animals, and flavoring them with natural, homegrown spices.

Once upon a time, we didn't need a multibillion-dollar beverage industry to keep us hydrated. We didn't need professional flavorists to formulate our drinks. Nor did we have to choose from what seems like an endless array of options. Beverages were simple, few, and WAMP; beers, milk, and herbal teas (also known as tisanes) were made at home or found locally. We weren't *buying* beverages when we got thirsty. We were drawing them from wells, milking them from animals, and flavoring them with unadulterated, homegrown spices.

Today's beverages are nothing like the liquids our species survived on (and thrived on) for tens of thousands of years. There were no nectars, coolers, or spritzers. There were just liquids that kept us alive and well.

This Reset will reveal an inconvenient truth: When it comes to the way we drink, nearly all the beverages we buy are completely *unnecessary to our lives*. "Beverages," for all intents and purposes, are a complete and utter sham.

With this Reset I am asking you to rethink your drink and start craving—and making—tastier and healthier beverages in your life.

Raise Your Glass to the Past: What We Need to Know About The Original Six Beverages

Water, animal milk, beer, wine, tea, and coffee. These six drinks made up humankind's original beverage industry. For generations, these nourishing WAMP drinks were perfectly suited for us. No flavorings, all simply made, and no food processing hoopla.

The first superheroes of the beverage world were good old-fashioned water and mother's breast milk. Until roughly 9000 BC, humans drank nothing else—no Vitaminwater, no Gatorade, no Jamba Juice, no apple juice, no Arizona Iced Tea, no Red Bull, no twenty-ounce Diet Coke.

At this time, researchers believe humans started consuming animal milk—most likely from sheep, not cows, and not pasteurized nor homogenized—quite different from the milk we drink today in those big, plastic gallon jugs and cartons.

We also discovered fermented drinks: beer and wine. They were a boon not so much for their inebriating effects but to help us avoid death. As we were transforming from hunter-gatherers to farming and pastoral communities, concentrated areas of feces and other wastes began to threaten safe water supplies, so in order to avoid harmful pathogens, we needed an alternative. Beer was the perfect solution, since the process of fermenting killed off any infectious agents. Beer was so beloved in ancient Egypt that it was consumed daily and was a common offering to the gods. Not merely a thirst-quencher, beer contained vital minerals and vitamins. It was the original health drink, though nothing like the pasteurized, highly processed brews we consume today.

Tea, the purported drink of Confucius, derives from the *Camellia sinensis* plant. Humans started drinking it around 2700 BC, when, legend has it, a tea leaf blew into Chinese emperor Shen Nung's cup of boiling water. Tea is one the world's oldest forms of natural caffeine and has been cherished by monks for centuries for its ability to imbue a sense of relaxed focus—a state critical to effective mediation. The ceremony of taking tea has been an intimate and celebrated part of human life throughout the ages in China, Japan, Russia, and England—a favorite drink of czars, queens, and emperors. Today, tea is the most popular drink in the world after water.

Coffee came next. The consumption of coffee beans is thought to have origins in Africa (supposedly the beans were eaten raw as early as the ninth century) sometime in the fourteenth century. It became a favorite drink of Muslim culture and coveted by the Ottoman Empire. Coffee didn't end up finding its way to America until after the Boston Tea Party in 1773, when colonists started to fish for an alternative source of caffeine after their symbolic obstruction of tea imports from the mother country.

Beverages Gone Wrong

Common Ingredients in Today's Processed Nonalcoholic Beverages

- Natural flavoring
- Malic acid
- Vitamin E
- Fumaric acid
- Sodium citrate
- Potassium citrate
- Potassium sorbate
- Potassium benzoate
- Aspartame
- Acesulfame
- Brominated vegetable oil
- Carob bean gum
- HFCS
- Modified food starch
- Sodium polyphosphates
- Glycerol ester of rosin

- Yellow #6
- Red #40
- Cream
- Maltodextrin
- Sucralose
- Chromium picolinate
- Purple sweet potato extractive
- L-Carnitine
- Caramel color
- Glucose
- Taurine
- Sorbic acid
- Reconstituted juice
- Juice concentrates
- Refined sugar

The Original Six Are Nixed

Unfortunately, over the past century, we've managed to threaten the sanctity of the original six. No longer are we drinking to to keep us alive, nourished, and hydrated. No longer does the deliciousness of beverages come from using all-natural processes.

Instead, most of what we drink today make us sip and gulp for the wrong reasons while filling our bodies with food additives and chemicals. On top of that, ready-to-drink teas, vitamin-enhanced quenchers, and every other processed drink out there are robbing our taste buds of the flavor our bodies really want to crave.

Soda Pop: The Big Kahuna

Not surprisingly, soda is one of the best examples of beverages going awry. Believe it or not, soda was never meant to be sweet, just bubbly. Thanks to the intrepid Romans, interest in the pure waters of naturally effervescent mineral springs led to a concerted effort on the part of British royalty (specifically King Charles II) to find a way to mimic these special liquids for medicinal and therapeutic purposes beginning in the seventeenth century. An English chap named Joseph Priestly is credited with inventing what we now call "soda" by using carbonation to create bubbles in 1772—the term "soda" is a reference to the bicarbonate of soda used to create the carbonation.

Soda was originally marketed to a public who wanted a virtually tasteless, sugar-free, therapeutic drink that had the health properties of natural mineral waters. It was first sold primarily at pharmacies.

It wasn't long, though, before additional ingredients such as wine, spices, sarsaparilla, ginger, and lemon were added—experiments by chemists. Around the mid-nineteenth century refined sugar was added to soda, making it sweet, once and for all. At the end of the century, sugar-toting Dr. Pepper, Coca-Cola, and Pepsi-Cola were invented—in 1885, 1886, and 1898 respectively.

If you take a look at Coca-Cola's original formulation, you'll notice just how much more processed modern Coke is than its predecessor. Coca-Cola's original recipe, invented by John Pemberton, called for caffeine citrate, fluid extract of coca leaves, real lime juice, real caramel, real cane sugar, real vanilla extract, and oils of cinnamon,

Ingredient Comparison: Sodas

Original WAMP Soda

- Carbonated water

Today's Processed Soda

- Carbonated water
- HFCS
- Citric acid
- Sodium benzoate
- Natural flavors
- Modified food starch
- Sodium polyphosphates
- Glycerol ester of rosin
- Yellow #6
- Brominated vegetable oil
- Red #40

- Potassium citrate
- Potassium sorbate
- Potassium benzoate
- Aspartame
- Acesulfame potassium
- Carob bean gum
- Caffeine
- Phosphoric acid
- Juice concentrates
- Refined sugar

nutmeg, and neroli. These were all ingredients that, for the most part, were WAMP, not made up in some laboratory.

Twist around a can of today's Coca-Cola and you'll find "Carbonated Water, High Fructose Corn Syrup, Caramel Color, Phosphoric Acid, Natural Flavors, Caffeine" on the label. Those aren't ingredients I can buy at the supermarket, and they definitely aren't WAMP.

Pulp Fiction: The Truth About Juice

Highly processed beverages that are useless to our bodies don't stop with soda pop. The sabotage of hydration goes on and on, with drinks that fall into categories like "fruit beverages," "functional drinks," "energy drinks," and "sports drinks." Even coffee and tea (of our original six) have been corrupted.

One of the biggest gimmicks when it comes to modern beverages is the application of the word "juice." You might be thinking that juice is as old as time—even wondering why it's not among the original six. Surely where there were oranges in history, there was orange juice. If our ancestors had grapes, they must have made grape juice, right? Truth is, we didn't start drinking what we now think of as a glass of juice until the sixteenth century, when, some scholars suggest, lemonade was created in medieval Egypt using wine, lemons, dates, and honey. We certainly know that carrying lime and lemon juice on ocean journeys was mandatory for British vessels in the nineteenth century by way of the Merchant Shipping Act of 1867. Yet, truth be told, we didn't start drinking what we now think of as juice en masse until the twentieth century.

> Juice has spawned several beverage subcategories such as "fruit juices" and "fruit cocktails." These drinks often contain almost no juice at all.

Another fact that puts things in perspective: The juicer wasn't even invented until the 1930s, and mainstream consumption of orange juice didn't start until the Florida citrus crisis in the 1950s. As with soda, the first juices were whole and minimally processed, and therefore relatively healthful. They were made fresh and consumed fresh—simply the squeezed juices extracted from fruits. Now, however, most juices—particularly the orange juice you find in the refrigerated section of your grocery store—are either made from concentrate or pasteurized (heated at extreme temperatures for short periods of time, which kills off vitamins, minerals, and enzymes) to ensure they can stay shelf-stable. They also contain additional sugars, flavorings, and other ingredients to make them palatable.

Juice has spawned several beverage subcategories such as "fruit juices" and "fruit cocktails," terms that describe any beverage that contains a blend of fruit juice and other ingredients. These drinks often contain almost *no juice at all*; for example, some Fuze drinks, a juice brand of Coca-Cola, contain just 5 percent juice. These beverages are all completely superfluous to our biological needs and perfect examples of the beverage industry taking us for a ride.

Ingredient Comparison: Juices

Original WAMP Juice

- 100 percent fresh-squeezed juice

Processed Fruit Juices, Fruit Cocktails, Nectars, Fruit Drinks

- Juice concentrates
- Cane sugar
- Citric acid
- Evaporated cane juice
- Natural flavors
- Sugar
- Ascorbic acid
- Aspartame
- Reconstituted fruit juices
- Vitamin E
- Fumaric acid
- Vitamin A palmitate

"Enhanced" Drinks and More

Sports drinks, performance drinks, and enhanced waters, have been dubbed "functional drinks," yet they don't provide much in the way of better functionality for the human body. They're really just another way to repackage simple drinks like plain water into liquids that are sweet and processed. As we learned in the chapter titled The Power of WAMP, the best way to obtain nutrients for our bodies is through WAMP foods, so no matter how much vitamin C, vitamin B, antioxidants, and other "immunity-boosting" ingredients these beverages claim to have, they'll never be able to deliver. Sure, some sports drinks can provide an electrolyte advantage, but most are still doused with stuff we don't need, namely sugar. Energy drinks are just another way to repackage the caffeine we could otherwise be getting from simply made tea and coffee into something that's entirely unneeded and not in concert with our biological make-up. There's no need for extra levels of caffeine that are products of food processing. In other words, Mother Nature didn't mean for us to be high on Red Bull.

Ready-to-drink teas, coffees, and espresso drinks have also been bastardized. We've been conditioned to think "coffee" means a caramel soy latte—a recipe which contains processed sweetened soy milk, food industry manufactured simple syrups, and dollops of whip cream—and Starbucks bottled Frappuccinos, which count sugar and maltodextrin as its key ingredients.

Tea drinks aren't any better. From bottled peach iced teas to diet green tea lemonades, one of the purest, healthiest drinks on Earth has been transformed into a sugar-spiked, watered-down corrupted version of its former self. Nearly 85 percent of the tea we drink in the United States today is processed, sweetened, and consumed iced, not hot.

Messing with Our Brain Chemistry

In 2010, the average American drank nearly sixty-four and a half gallons of carbonated sodas, fruit beverages, and sports, energy, and functional drinks—none of it necessary

---

Ingredient Comparison: Waters

WAMP Water

• Water

Processed Sports Drinks and Enhanced Waters

• Water

• Sucrose

• Citric acid

• Natural flavor

• Artificial flavor

• Salt

• Sodium citrate

• Monopotassium phosphate

• Sucralose

• Red #40

• Acesulfame potassium

• Sugar

• Gum arabic

• Potassium chloride

• Crystalline fructose

• Cane sugar

• Vitamin B5

• Vitamin B6

• Vitamin B12

• Magnesium lactate

Ingredient Comparison: Caffeinated Beverages

WAMP Tea and Coffee

- Water
- Tea leaves
- Coffee beans
- Minimal additions of milk and sugar

Processed Energy Drinks, Ready-to-Drink Tea, and Coffee Beverages

- Agave syrup
- Sucralose
- Citric acid
- Acesulfame potassium
- Natural flavors
- Sugar
- Sucralose
- Maltodextrine sugar
- Taurine
- Gum arabic
- Caramel color
- Potassium chloride
- Sodium hexametaphosphate
- Crystalline fructose
- Caffeine
- Cane sugar
- Inositol
- Vitamin B5
- Magnesium oxide
- Vitamin B6
- Cane sugar
- Vitamin B12
- HFCS
- Magnesium lactate

and none of it nourishing. This begs the question: Why in the world do we feel so compelled to sip sugary drinks ad nauseam when our biochemistry doesn't require it?

Beverages are no different than solid foods. As with processed sugary foods, processed sugary drinks exploit our innate weakness for sweetness. Our neurocircuitry zones in on the engineered sweetness in our drinks and wants more. A growing body of evidence has come to reveal that sugary beverages have the ability to hijack our brains in ways that promote addictive tendencies. In fact, some researchers have even compared their effects to that of drug addiction. When lab rats were subjected to sugar water every day, over time, they wanted more and more.

And not only do we want more iced teas, sodas, and juice drinks, we also end up wanting less of the healthy stuff—the original WAMP beverages our ancestors thrived on for hundreds of thousands of years. The flavors of sugar-spiked energy drinks and corn-syrup-doused soda make it exceedingly hard for us to enjoy the delectably bitter flavor of things like minimally processed black coffee and green tea. Even plain milk, which contains the naturally occurring sugar lactose, isn't sweet enough for us. We prefer sugary chocolate and strawberry versions.

Processed beverages also create something scientists call "hedonic thirst," whereby things like carbonation, color, flavor strength, and temperature, together with sugar, can be manipulated to "encourage drinking that is not necessarily linked to fluid needs." In other words, we fall prey to the fizziness that envelops our mouths, the bubbles that release when we pop the top, the added acids (e.g., phosphoric acid) that impart just the right flavor when we take a sip, and the refreshing taste of an ice-cold beverage on a hot summer day. They all make us want more. They lure us, excite us, and seduce us into buying and drinking, even when we're not feeling thirsty.

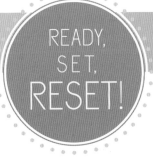

It's obvious that our relationship with beverages has gone awry: They're not WAMP, they're everywhere, and we're needlessly dependent on them. But reading about them isn't enough. It's time to make a big change to our lives, and with this Reset, that's exactly what we will do! To effectively change how we drink, we can't just learn about the problem, we need to act to solve it—we need to experience anew. In this part of the Reset, we're going to touch, taste, and discover how healthy, WAMP beverages are chock-full of flavor—more flavor than you can imagine.

In fact, when we take back the power of beverage-making from food manufacturers, we experience deliciousness on a whole new level. The flavor in many of the drinks you're going to make will take your taste buds to a territory of temptation you may never have thought possible. This is no bland Reset!

In fact, plain water isn't even part of this plan. These drink recipes are inspired by the past, and if we look back in history, we find plenty of examples—especially from ancient Egypt and ancient China—where plain water was flavored with delectable and healthy ingredients— fragrant fresh herbs, orange peels, and peppermint and licorice roots. Spices such as cardamom, and flowers such as

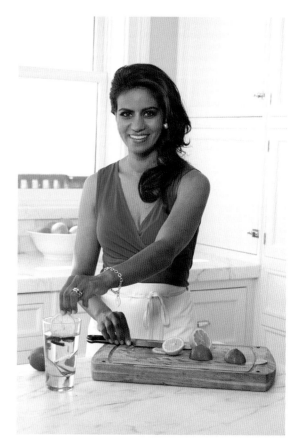

chamomile and jasmine, have also historically been used in water to impart sweet, savory, and spicy flavors and sensual aromas. We can do this too. Getting excited?

There are millions of ways to stay deliciously hydrated without succumbing to processed beverages. We just need to learn how! That's what we'll do in the next seventy-two hours.

Instructions

For the next three days you will abstain from *all processed and sweetened, store-bought beverages,* with the exception of plain coconut water, fresh-squeezed juices, black coffee, unsweetened hot and/or iced tea, and plain milk (low-fat, skim, and whole are all fine; choose milk from grass-fed sources if possible).

Root Beer

Did you know that root beer, an all-American favorite, was originally WAMP? Before mass manufacturers took over, it was home-brewed and consisted of a variety of plant materials, such as sarsaparilla root, sassafras root, dandelion root, ginger root, birch bark, wild cherry bark, wintergreen bark, allspice, juniper berries, vanilla bean, cinnamon, and molasses or cane sugar.

Any beverage that includes artificial or "zero-calorie" sugars is off-limits. I know this may pose a challenge to your routine, especially if you rely on sweet, caffeinated beverages like soda or energy drinks. But remember, it's just three days. You can do this!

In exchange for your abstinence from processed drinks, you now have the opportunity to indulge in some wildly flavorful, WAMP substitutes. Below I've included six WAMP beverage recipes you can make at any time throughout this period. You can attempt some or all, but you must try *at least three recipes* over the course of this Reset. You can drink as many servings as you wish. There are no limitations, but keep in mind that moderation is the best policy, especially with regard to the two caloric drinks—the Lemon-Lime Soda and Fresh-Squeezed OJ—for which you should plan to have no more than two servings per day. You'll also notice that some of the recipes call for additional sweeteners, yet all of these sweeteners are unrefined and, as such, are WAMP ingredients (check back to the Sugar Reset chapter for a review of WAMP sugar).

Because we spend so much time outside our homes and the majority of the recipes below are much easier to make in the comfort of your own kitchen, you'll need to plan accordingly. If you're sure you can't get through the workday by drinking the acceptable drinks I mentioned above, plan to make a recipe or two before you go to work, and bring it along with you. For example, if you hate plain water, you might want to make the Zen Water and bring it with you in a thermos.

For some, caffeine may pose a challenge. You won't be able to get your fix from caramel lattes, Coke, Pepsi, or bottled sugary iced teas during this Reset. I won't lie:

Detox

By cutting back on caffeinated and sugary drinks, you may experience side effects: Slight headaches, change in mood, and waning energy may challenge you. Don't give up! Do your best to persevere. These symptoms alone prove how important this Reset is. Remember, it takes time to transition into more subtle, simple, and healthier drinks like green tea. Be prepared, and know that this Reset is cleansing you of toxins that are harmful to your body and brain. It's just three days—you can do this! To alleviate any potential symptoms, try keeping yourself well hydrated: Coconut water (the tastiest kind comes from a young coconut, and can be found these at places like Whole Foods Market) is a wonderful choice for this, as well as fresh-squeezed juices and the Zen Water recipe below. You can also try staying active, taking brisk walks while breathing deeply—both help to boost energy levels and your immune system. Hop over to the gym, or do yoga. In the end, you'll want to be easy on yourself and take time out for your body to relax and unwind as much as possible while you do this Reset.

It's not easy to make an abrupt change to your caffeine needs, but with the recipes below and your ability to drink *pure* coffee and tea, you have some excellent alternatives. When you're drinking coffee during these three days, stick with the highest-quality brew you can find with the highest-quality milk and the least refined sugars you can find. This means that you may want to track down a local coffee shop that either roasts beans in house or can tell you where and when their beans were roasted as well as the origin of the beans—all signs of good quality. Try plain lattes and cappuccinos (just espresso and good-quality milk) and plain black coffee (using an individual-cup drip or French press brewing techniques, for example) if you can. Like WAMP chocolate, a good cup of black coffee should be wildly flavorful–smooth and beautifully fragrant with hints of several taste and aroma notes (e.g., delicate, fruity, nutty, chocolaty). If you can't tolerate it without some form of sweetener, tuck a small container of whole-cane sugar or coconut-palm sugar in your bag before you leave the house. With tea, do the same: Drink plain tea (tea bag or loose-leaf), and if you need to sweeten it, use WAMP sugar crystals or, better yet, a little honey and lemon—this fragrant combination is best for black teas. You can also choose to make the iced tea recipe below.

TIPS & TOOLS for EACH DAY

Changing the way you drink for three days is a revolutionary act. What you'll be tasting, smelling, seeing, and learning will awaken and inspire. Here are some tips to guide you on your way.

Day One

Welcome to the first day of this potentially life-altering seventy-two-hour journey! If you usually depend on processed beverages to start your day—a syrup-filled vanilla latte, coffee drowned with table sugar and/or a nondairy processed creamer, a diet soda—you'll come across your first challenge right away. Take this opportunity to make the Moroccan Mint Tea, the Jasmine Green Tea recipe, or go for pure coffee. All of these will give you a kick of caffeine, but in a WAMP way.

If you choose to make the jasmine tea, take your time with it, making sure you follow the directions to a T (pun intended!). Brewing loose-leaf tea is a science that demands precision and yields sensational rewards. Make sure you follow the brewing instructions perfectly time so as not to impart too much bitterness to your drink. And when you're ready to take the first sip, savor the wonderful aromas that envelop your nose and mouth as you bring the cup to your lips. Jasmine has a sweet, narcotic scent that is sophisticated and inspiring. I chose to include this tea here because it has been savored and enjoyed by the Chinese for generations. It's a beverage that one should try at least once in one's lifetime.

Tea Party

Add these to herbal or black teas for extraordinary flavor:

- Lemongrass
- Cinnamon sticks
- Anise seed
- Fennel seed
- Fresh peppermint leaves
- Fresh lemon verbena leaves
- Manuka honey (the most nutrient-dense raw honey on the planet)

As a side note, to get the most caffeine and best flavor from a cup of tea, opt for a black, loose-leaf tea. Loose-leaf tea tends to be made of whole, high-quality tea leaves as opposed to tea bags made of cut leaves that don't offer the same superior flavor. If you can't find loose-leaf tea, buy a bag of high-quality black—Assam or Ceylon are two flavorful options. (Note: English Breakfast, Irish Breakfast, etc. are blended teas and as such are harder to judge for quality). These do well accompanied by a squeeze of lemon and a drip of honey.

If you want to make a fantastic cup of coffee, use the freshest, highest-quality ground coffee (or grind your own beans), and brew it using a French press, a paper filter, or a similar tool. As with high-quality loose-leaf tea, there's really no substitute for the flavor of fresh-ground, high-quality coffee prepared correctly. Having coffee prepared in this way will make a cup from Dunkin' Donuts taste washed-out.

If instead you want to buy a hot cup of tea or coffee at the coffee shop or snag some from your office coffeemaker, add nothing more than a bit of high-quality milk and/ or an unrefined sweetener. Remember: You may want to bring some unrefined sugar crystals in a pouch along with you for the day.

It's best to try teas and coffees without any additional flavoring at first in order to

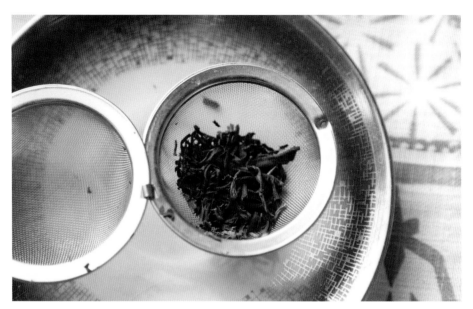

Black tea leaves after steeping

experience the authentic flavor of each. Although it is surprising to most people, tea and coffee—just like chocolate—are naturally bitter. We should aim to enjoy them in this way. And if we can't drink them plain, we should make sure that what we do add to them—cream, honey, sweeteners, etc.—doesn't drown out their authentic flavor but rather enhances it.

As a general rule, as you continue moving through the day—and the Reset as a whole—quench your thirst with water, get your energy boost from fresh-squeezed juices and tea or coffee, and satisfy your sweet tooth with WAMP foods, not sugary beverages.

At lunchtime, instead of an iced soda or iced tea with your meal, try iced water or iced sparkling water with a squeeze of lemon, lime, or orange. You'll be astonished how much of a kick you get from this simple concoction. Just the scent of fresh lemon is invigorating.

As you work your way into the afternoon and evening, keep experimenting with teas, both caffeinated and herbal. Oftentimes, we reach for caloric drinks when we're anxious or uneasy. Teas do a wonderful job of calming our nerves and getting us into a Zen state without any preservatives, additives, or calories. Look for teas that are whole and loose-leaf.

Over the years, I've found that if I'm not thirsty and not hungry, yet there's still *something* I'm after, a hot cup of tea usually gets me back to center. There's something about the aroma, the feeling of holding a warm teacup in your hands, and the sensation of hot liquid on the lips that automatically soothes, uplifts, and relaxes.

Tonight, you might want to try the Zen Water. It is very easy to make, and you can put your pitcher right into the fridge so it's chilled and ready for you to enjoy tomorrow morning.

If you're a milk drinker or you enjoy milk in your tea, stop by a natural foods store to buy grass-fed milk. After experiencing this kind of milk, you'll never want to go back to the old kind. Believe me, the taste is beyond extraordinary: creamier, richer, and perfectly sweet. And this milk is more nutrient-dense than other varieties.

As you finish your day, take a mental note of how little is required to make water taste better: herbs, fruits, citrus.

Day Two

Good morning! Now that you've gotten your feet wet with this Reset, today you can relax a little.

This morning, try to making the WAMP OJ recipe. When I first did this a few years back, it blew my mind. It seems embarrassingly simple. You cut an orange in half and squeeze out its juices using a reamer or your own two hands, and drink. Sometimes simple is brilliant!

Fruit juices—particularly orange juice—have been imagined by the food industry to be a complicated beverage that we *need* to buy from a grocery store. What you'll find is that the best OJ requires no food processing at all and is a million times more flavorful than anything you'd buy in a carton or plastic bottle. That's because it's fresh and minimally processed. Next time you're at the grocery store, make it a point to check the ingredient list of a pasteurized orange juice. Note that it's been heated to kill bacteria (pasteurized), which sacrifices flavor, and it won't tell you *when* the juice was harvested. Was it two weeks ago, a few months ago? In other words, it's not as "fresh-squeezed" as you might think.

Over the course of the day, think about juice overall—apple juices, grapefruit juices, vegetable juices—and compare store-bought kinds to fresh-squeezed alternatives. By scanning labels, you'll see that most are made of concentrated and reconstituted juices (juice that's been meddled with after its been extracted). Some even contain lab-created flavorings to make up for any loss in flavor due to processing.

Today, perhaps on your lunch break, seek out a fresh-squeezed juice purveyor close to you—maybe a local juice bar or health food spot—and compare this kind of juice with the juice drinks or bottled juices you're used to. You'll realize right off the bat that the fresh-squeezed juice is nothing short of magnificent. It looks better and even smells better! Actually, most processed bottled juices and juice drinks don't have an aroma at all. Where did the natural scents go?

I must point out, however, that when you buy fresh juice that's been made using a machine juicer, you are losing out on all the beautiful fiber and other nutrients that go to waste in the process. Remember, juice isn't a whole food. So I recommend you drink juice only when you feel you need a boost, or simply in moderation.

As you work your way through the rest of the day, consider how unnecessary it is for juice drinks and iced teas to be sweetened with refined and processed sugars. All this does is manipulate our innate craving for sweetness. *There's simply no good reason for sugar to be in our beverages.*

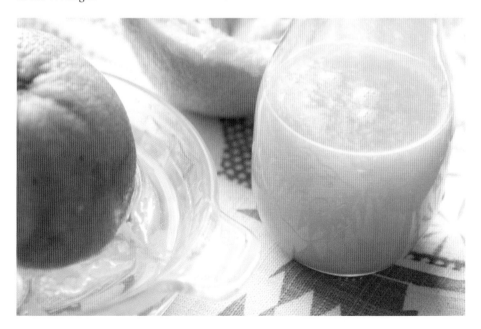

Tonight, try making the iced-tea recipe if you're so inclined. It's an easy one and perfect for those who enjoy bottled iced-tea beverages. It's yet another skill to have under your belt as you try to pry away beverage-making from the clutches of the food-processing industry. One interesting fact to keep in mind is that we didn't start drinking iced tea until the early twentieth century. Before this, we'd only enjoyed hot tea.

Day Three

You're almost there! On this third day, do more investigating. If you have a few minutes free while you're waiting for the subway, take a stroll over to the newsstand or bodega, or any establishment that sells beverages, and scan the ingredient lists: How many words can you pronounce? How many weird-sounding line items do you see? Why is what we drink as much or even more processed than what we eat?

While you go about your day today, ask friends, colleagues, and family about what they usually drink. Do they think about the processing that goes into most beverages? Do they feel it's as important to think about what we drink as what we eat? Do they know how much flavor they may be missing by drinking processed beverages?

Share your newfound enlightenment. Even share your recipes and your tricks for making water and orange juice taste better. You'll be stunned by how much more you learn just by chatting with others.

When you get home today, you may want try the remaining beverages: the Blackberry Lime Rickey and Lemon-Lime Soda. Both of these drinks are meant to mimic sweet-tasting carbonated processed beverages like 7UP. As you're making these simple recipes, notice the amount of flavor that comes from items like blackberries and herbs. Realize that fresh, WAMP ingredients yield so much more flavor—the core truth that resonates throughout every chapter and recipe in this book.

Last, if you have time today, stroll through the beverage aisle at your neighborhood supermarket. I guarantee, if you haven't done this in a while, it's a jaw-dropping experience. Beverages have come to take up hundreds of feet of shelf space. You'll find innumerable varieties of iced teas, juice drinks, juice pouches, coffee drinks, and energy drinks—all processed and completely unnecessary to our health. Read the labels, read the ingredient lists, and fully take in this reality.

Recommended WAMP Store-Bought Beverage Brands

Bottled Tea Drinks
- Ito En Tea's Tea
  (any unsweetened variety)
- Ito En Tea Shots
- Ito En Oi Ocha
- Tejava

Flavored Water
- Herbal Water
- Montauk Beverage Works

Miscellaneous
- GT's Kombucha

Tea Bags and Loose-Leaf
- Republic of Tea
- Rishi Tea
- Numi Tea

Grass-Fed Milk and Cream*
- Straus Family Creamery
- Organic Valley

* Check with your local purveyors and farmers markets. The best-tasting milk always comes from close to home.

Your accomplishments with this Reset are monumental. Bask in the knowledge that you can now replicate many of the decaffeinated sodas you buy at the grocery store in the comfort of your own home. Take pride in knowing that you don't have to rely on the beverage industry to enjoy delicious, carbonated refreshments. Delight in the idea that you now know each and every ingredient that goes into what you sip and gulp. What an accomplishment!

After the Reset

In only seventy-two hours, this Reset has awakened you to just how unhealthily we're drinking and, maybe more important, how much we're missing in terms of flavor! We've been sipping nutrient-poor, super-sweet drinks with compromised taste.

But now, you have a whole new set of tools and facts that can help you to drink healthier beverages for the rest of your life. With this Reset, you've discovered recipes that you can continue to make and enjoy, and modify to your liking. You've got a brand new

YOUR BEVERAGE RESET GROCERY LIST

- [ ] 2 organic lemons
- [ ] 1 organic Granny Smith apple or similar apple
- [ ] 1 navel orange
- [ ] 3–4 oranges for juicing
- [ ] 2 sprigs fresh thyme or 1 sprig rosemary
- [ ] Frozen or fresh blackberries
- [ ] 1 sprig basil
- [ ] 2 limes
- [ ] 20 oz club soda or sparkling water
- [ ] Pure Grade A maple syrup
- [ ] Loose-leaf black tea
- [ ] 1 sprig fresh mint
- [ ] Loose-leaf jasmine green tea

understanding of how to choose the best drinks for you and how to navigate your everyday life when it comes to hydrating yourself (to get you started, I've included my favorite store-bought WAMP beverage brands on page 211).

With this Reset you've found more flavor in coffee and tea. Perhaps now you're willing to fork over more money for a single, high-quality cup of joe than for several of the kind you've been drowning in refined sugar and creamer for the last ten years. And depending on the sensitivity of your taste buds prior to undergoing this Reset, you may have come away realizing that the drinks you were used to are now too sweet for your liking.

Going forward, it will be easy to permanently integrate the rules of this Reset into your everyday life. If you do so, overtime, sodas and sweet drinks will start to give you sugar rushes or headaches, and will likely taste too sweet for your palate. Don't be surprised if you become much more reliant on water. As your taste buds adjust, you'll prefer teas and coffees plain.

If you choose not to quit processed drinks completely, apply the 80/20 Rule. If you can limit 80 percent of your drinks to WAMP beverages, you'll be golden!

Jasmine Green Tea

For those unfamiliar with the flavor of green tea or those who find it too bitter, this kind of green tea offers a more palatable alternative as the beautiful, strong aroma and flavor of jasmine offsets the bitterness and at the same time, captivates the senses. These teas are made by layering fresh jasmine flowers among tea leaves, not by spraying the leaves in any way. This authentic, ages old type of scented tea needs only three minutes of infusion. When you are done, the same leaves can be infused for a second cup. The key to enjoying this recipe is to find the highest-quality jasmine green tea you can. I like Jasmine Pearl loose-leaf tea from a company called Rishi Tea. You can find their products at Whole Foods and other stores or online.

SERVES: 1
TOTAL TIME: 5 MINUTES

INGREDIENTS
* 1 tbsp loose leaf jasmine green tea
* 8 oz filtered cold water

PROCEDURE

1. Place tea leaves in an infuser of choice (mesh ball, bag, etc.) and place in serving teacup or glass.

2. Bring water to a boil, wait a minute, then pour it over the tea leaves. Let it steep for exactly three minutes—no longer or your tea will become too bitter.

3. Remove the tea infuser or strain the tea, keeping the tea leaves for another infusion.

Citrus Zen Water

BEVERAGE RESET RECIPE

This recipe is a spa visit in a pitcher! It makes drinking water fragrant, sensual, and uplifting. Use this as your go-to daily beverage.

SERVES: 6–8
TOTAL TIME: 5 MINUTES

INGREDIENTS

- 1/2 organic lemon, washed, and thinly sliced, discarding end segment
- 1/2 organic granny smith apple, cored, halved, and thinly sliced
- Several very thin (1/8 inch thick) slices organic navel orange
- 6–8 c cold filtered water
- 2 sprigs fresh thyme or 1 stem rosemary (optional)

PROCEDURE

1. Place all ingredients into a large pitcher and let sit at room temperature or you if prefer it chilled, put in refrigerator for at least 10 minutes.

2. Pour into your favorite glass with or without ice and enjoy.

Notes:

- To keep it longer, strain all ingredients (over time, they will make the water bitter) from the pitcher and store it in the fridge for days.

- You need not use all ingredients to make beautifully flavored water. Just oranges or herbs will do the trick.

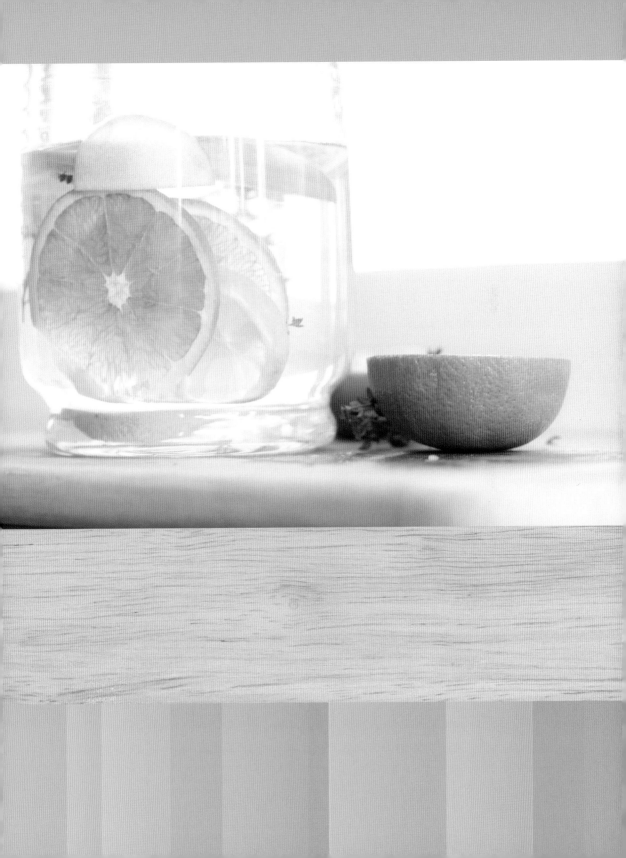

No Sugar Blackberry Lime Rickey (Virgin)

BEVERAGE RESET RECIPE

This über-flavorful beverage will make you rethink sugary drinks for good! Fresh basil, sweet blackberries, and kick of acidity and sour from lime juice make this non-alcoholic drink a WAMP beverage masterpiece.

SERVES: 1
TOTAL TIME: 12 MINUTES

INGREDIENTS

- 5 fresh or frozen blackberries
- 5 fresh basil leaves, torn or roughly chopped
- juice of 1/4 lime, keeping wedge
- 12 oz club soda or sparkling water
- Ice (optional)

PROCEDURE

1. If using frozen blackberries, allow them to defrost at room temperature or defrost them in a microwave. Place berries at the bottom of a glass along with basil. Using a spoon or blunted object, crush (muddle) the berries and basil. Add 8 oz club soda and allow to marinate for 10 minutes.

2. Strain, discarding the basil and blackberry portions. Add remaining club soda and add juice of lime and drop the wedge into the glass. Enjoy immediately with or without ice!

Lemon-Lime Soda

BEVERAGE RESET RECIPE

I created this recipe as a substitute for sodas. You'll find that a Sprite or 7UP can't compare! Add lemon or lime peel for a beautiful visual accent and gorgeous aroma.

SERVES: 1
TOTAL TIME: 5 MINUTES

INGREDIENTS

- 2 tsp lime juice
- 2 tsp lemon juice
- 2 tsp pure Grade A maple syrup
- 8 oz sparkling water (ex. club soda, sparkling mineral water)
- Lemon/Lime rind or slices for garnish (optional)
- Ice (optional)

PROCEDURE

1. Add all ingredients to your favorite glass and stir to combine. Add ice if you prefer. Enjoy serious refreshment!

Moroccan Mint Tea

This recipe is inspired by an original Moroccan recipe. Fresh mint is the perfect compliment to black tea while maple syrup—a WAMP sweetener—adds just the right amount of sweet to balance the overall flavor.

SERVES: 1
TOTAL TIME: 5 MINUTES

INGREDIENTS
- 2 tsp to 1 tbsp loose leaf black tea
- 6 fresh mint leaves (or about 1 full sprig)
- Filtered cold water
- 1 1/2 tsp pure grade A maple syrup (optional)

Note: Instead of maple syrup, you can use any minimally refined sweetener of your choice—see page 59 for a list.

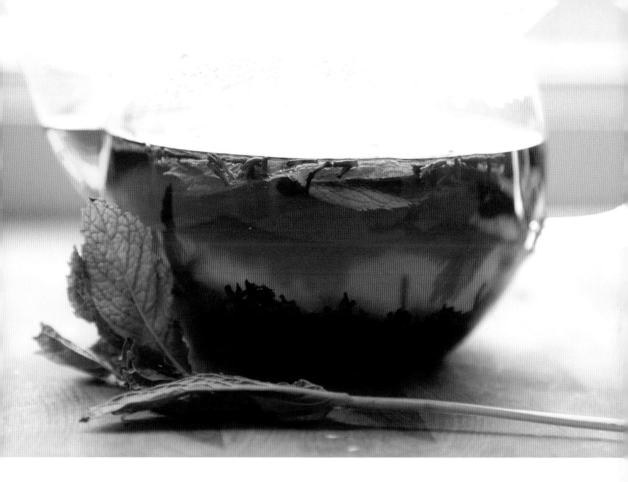

PROCEDURE

1. Place tea leaves in an infuser of choice (mesh ball, bag, etc.) and place in a serving teacup or glass along with mint leaves (throw in the entire sprig if you wish).

2. Bring water to a boil, remove from heat, and pour over tea leaves and mint. Let steep for 4 to 5 minutes—no longer or your tea will become too bitter.

3. At the 4 to 5 minute mark, remove the tea infuser or strain tea, keeping tea leaves for another infusion. At this point you may either discard the mint leaves or leave them in the liquid.

4. Add syrup, stir and enjoy your hot cup while meditating in peaceful bliss.

WAMP OJ

This is hands-down the easiest, healthiest, and most nourishing way to enjoy orange juice! By using a handheld or tabletop reamer as opposed to a machine juicer, you keep more fiber in your juice, which adds to its flavor as well as its nutrient properties.

SERVES: 1–2
TOTAL TIME: 5 MINUTES

INGREDIENTS

- 3 large Valencia or Navel oranges
  (or another large orange suitable for juicing), cut in half

PROCEDURE

1. Using a hand held citrus reamer or flat tabletop citrus reamer, squeeze as much juice as you can from each orange half. Pour juice into your favorite glass and enjoy immediately.

Note: Your juice will be at the height of its flavor when it is first squeezed. You can store it in the fridge with a tight lid for two to three days.

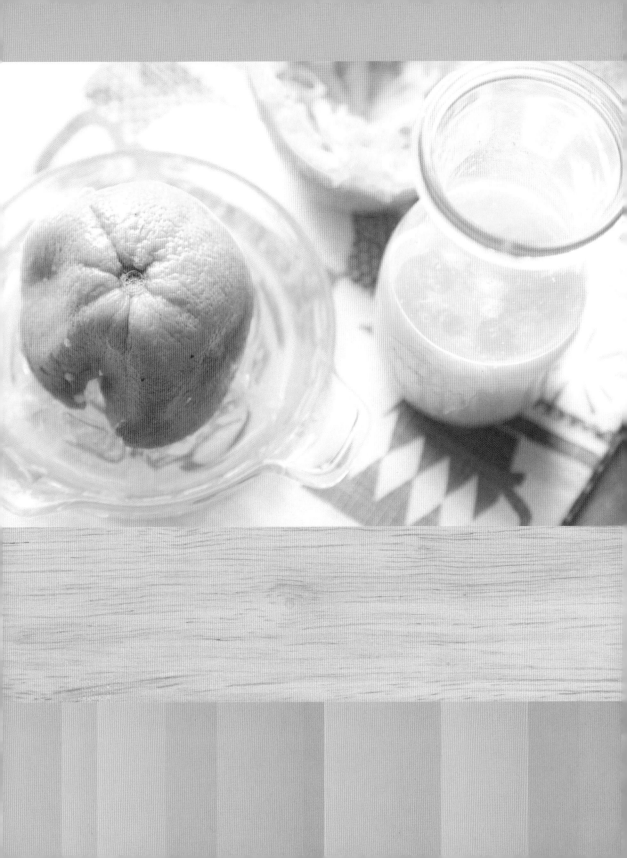

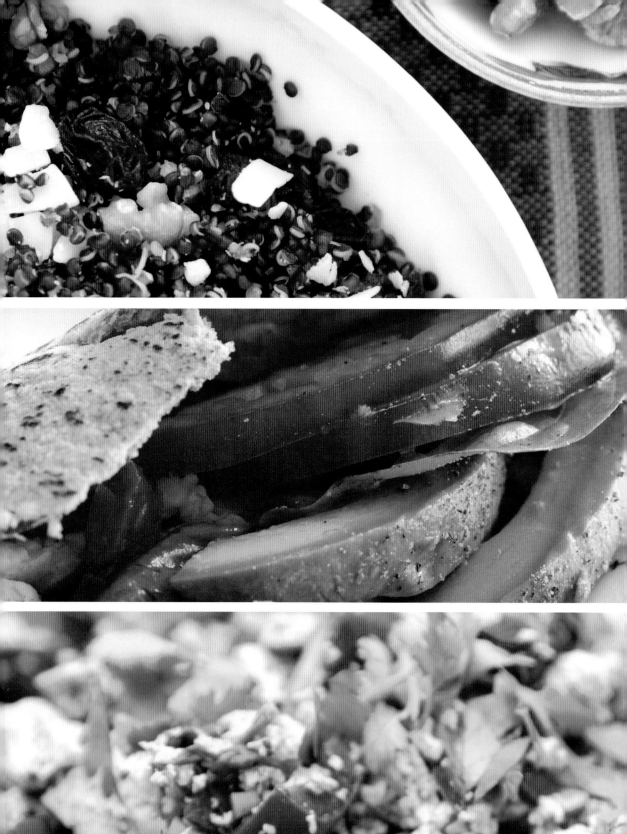

Breakfast
RESET

Deceptive and dishonest. That's how I describe the standard morning meal we all call "breakfast." Although this morning ritual might seem innocent to you, it's got "guilty" written all over it. If there's one meal of the day that we need to reset, it's this one.

Breakfast is like a powerful dictator: It's formed a monopoly on food that holds many of us hostage between the hours of 6:00 AM and 10:00 AM. Think about it: Breakfast is the only meal of the day that seems to have strict expectations about what we can and can't eat in the morning: Cold cereal, hot cereal, bagels with cream cheese, toast and eggs, coffee and doughnuts, a vanilla latte with a blueberry scone all get the green light. On the weekends: waffles, omelets, and French toast are our headliners. The roster of breakfast foods never really changes, and hasn't for decades. Who made these rules?

With more than 60 percent of our breakfast menu anchored in refined sugar and refined flour, not only are we being limited by our choices, but we're being forced to eat

> ## Morning Dessert
>
> About 60 percent of the foods we eat for breakfast—cereals, bagels, pancakes, pastries, etc.—are made primarily of wheat flour and refined sugar—so much flour and sugar that we might as well be calling our breakfast "dessert."

food that's not WAMP. All those cinnamon scones, cranberry muffins, boxed cereals, instant oats, bagels, and syrup-drenched pancakes are highly processed, created using refined sugar and refined wheat flour, the same two ingredients that go into cakes, cookies, and pies.

Processed wheat plus processed sugar? Yup, that's usually what's for breakfast. Not quite a wholesome, nourishing way to start the day, now, is it? No matter how much we might think what we're eating for breakfast is healthy and delicious, here's the truth: We can do a lot better. Today's breakfast foods are not living up to their potential, in terms of nutrition or flavor. Bagels with cream cheese, flaked cereal, strawberry waffles, and all the rest of the wheat-plus-sugar-based breakfast foods that have become the norm on millions of breakfast tables across the country aren't as tasty or satisfying as they could be.

It's time for this meal to be less restrictive, more delectable, and more WAMP. It's time to experience breakfast afresh. That's what this Reset is all about. We will turn breakfast upside down and inside out. By experimenting with breakfast foods made from WAMP ingredients and taking cues from the way others around the world eat breakfast, we will reboot the morning meal.

Buying Breakfast: What We Need to Know

These days, restaurant chains' breakfast offerings consist of everything from cinnamon scones to chocolate croissants to "wholesome" alternatives like oatmeal, fruit parfaits, and multigrain bagels. If you do a minute of digging into their ingredient lists, you'll find one common thread: Wheat flour and some type of added sugar are *never* missing. And all of it is processed food. For example, an oatmeal offering from a major fast-food chain features three different types of added sugars: dextrose, glucose, and evaporated cane juice. An ingredients list for a multigrain bagel at Dunkin' Donuts starts off with "wheat flour," and "sugar" comes in third, fourth, fifth, and second to last:

Enriched Wheat Flour (Wheat Flour, Niacin, Reduced Iron, Thiamin Mononitrate, Riboflavin, Folic Acid), Water, **Sugar**, Sugar-Infused Wild Blueberries (Blueberry, **High-Fructose Corn Syrup**, Water, Glycerol, Safflower Oil, Citric Acid, Calcium Lactate, Potassium Sorbate [Preservative], Natural Blueberry Flavors), Craisins (**Sugar**, Cranberries, Blueberry Juice from Concentrate, Grape Juice Concentrate, Sunflower Oil), Yeast, Wheat Gluten, Degermed Yellow Corn Meal, Salt, Malt Extract, Natural Blueberry Flavor, Natural Ferment Flavor (Cultured Wheat and Wheat-Malt Flours, Vinegar, Salt), Blueberries, Dough Conditioner (Malted Barley Flour, Enzymes, **Dextrose**), Soy (Trace).

Breakfast foods we buy at the grocery store—cereals, pancake mix, and apple-cinnamon instant oats—aren't any better. A leisurely stroll down the cereal aisle of your neighborhood supermarket is a flour-plus-sugar party. You'll find that almost every ingredient list on the most popular boxed cereals begins with the words "wheat flour," with added sugars trailing not far behind. Although not wheat-based, most instant oats packages come guaranteed with sweetness too. Even breakfast foods served hot on a plate—either by us or a short-order cook—such as pancakes and waffles, are made with packaged wheat-flour mixes. Here, the refined added sugar comes from their partner-in-crime, pancake syrup. You might as well call pancake syrup "pancake corn syrup" because that's more or less what it's made of. Here's the ingredient list from a leading pancake syrup brand:

Corn Syrup, **High Fructose Corn Syrup**, Water, Cellulose gum, Caramel color, salt, sodium benzoate and sorbic acid (preservatives), artificial and natural flavors, sodium hexametaphosphate.

Standard Breakfast Foods	Refined Sugars	Refined Wheat Flour
Boxed cereal	√	√
French toast with syrup	√	√
Multigrain bagel	√	√
Doughnut	√	√
Frozen toaster waffle	√	√
Blueberry scone	√	√
Bran muffin	√	√
Apple-cinnamon instant oatmeal	√	√

Scones, muffins, and pastries featured behind glass in almost every coffee-shop chain in America are also stellar examples of how our breakfast offerings have become defined by flour and sugar. Take a vanilla-frosted scone from a major coffeehouse chain as an example. Apart from the fact that this little scone has more than thirty-five ingredients (seriously, thirty-five), you'll notice that flour and added sugars dominate:

Enriched unbleached wheat flour (wheat flour, malted barley flour, niacin, reduced iron, thiamine mononitrate, riboflavin, folic acid), vanilla-bean glaze (**sugar**, water, **fructose**, contains 2 percent or less of the following: **corn syrup**, gum arabic, **honey**, potassium sorbate [preservative], agar, vanilla-bean seeds, citric acid, pectin, natural flavor, mono and diglycerides, locust bean gum), heavy cream, **sugar**, unsalted butter, whole eggs, soybean oil, baking powder (sodium acid pyrophosphate, sodium bicarbonate, cornstarch, monocalcium phosphate), nonfat dry milk, water, soy lecithin, **invert syrup**, natural vanilla flavor (vanilla bean, maltodextrin), salt, ground vanilla bean, xanthan gum.

This kind of breakfast food is strategically engineered to make us buy more of it, and less of everything else. As with cookies and ice cream, we are unfairly lured.

Hale and Hearty

What happened to that hearty American breakfast? Not too long ago, the average American breakfast was completely different—more WAMP, less sweet, more satisfying.

Processed wheat plus processed sugar? Yup, that's usually what's for breakfast. No matter how much we might think what we're eating for breakfast is delicious, here's the truth: We can do a lot better.

Pancakes and Syrup

A couple hundred years ago, breakfast cereals in a box didn't exist. Everything was made from scratch, mainly at home. Not much came out of a package or from a short order cook.

The pancakes of early America were much more WAMP than the pancakes you get today at IHOP or even a fancy brunch spot. Instead of wheat pancakes, early Americans ate buckwheat ("buckwheats") and cornmeal pancakes ("Indian cakes")—from flour ground at home. Incidentally, buckwheat—an ancient plant related to rhubarb—is gluten-free and contains many more nutrients, vitamins, and minerals when ground into flour than does wheat.

The first commercially sold, prepared, and packaged pancake "mix" was Aunt Jemima. But even in the late 1890s, it was made of a variety of flours: wheat, corn, and sometimes rye and rice. Now it's all just refined wheat.

In colonial times, pancake syrup wasn't made of corn syrup. It was 100 percent WAMP. Early settlers used pure maple syrup straight from the trees, likely a discovery by the Native Americans.

Muffins and Scones

The original muffins and scones were also worlds apart from their modern incarnations. For starters, neither was made with sugar like the raspberry-, cinnamon-, and blueberry-glazed scones we get today in little crinkly paper bags, with our morning lattes and cappuccinos. The first muffins were simple: a food made from bread dough but shaped differently. In England, muffins were toasted, buttered, and served with jam. What a world away from today's sugar-infused lemon poppy seed and reduced-fat bran muffins. Same goes for scones. The original scone, a traditional food of the Scottish, Irish, and English, was designed to be savory and even a bit sour. It was made of buttermilk, sour milk, or sour cream and wheat or barley meal, and also served hot and buttered.

Breakfast Pastry

Traditional brioche, croissants, and other breakfast baked goods made of butter, flour, and eggs were first made as foods of luxury, available only to the elite and wealthy. Apparently, the Austrian-born queen of France Marie Antoinette, wife of King Louis XIV, requested a croissant every day. But that we now treat goods of the patisserie as if they were nothing more than the standard sidekick to a hot cup of joe must tell us something. And the original croissant was not pumped full of chocolate, as it is today.

Cold Boxed Cereal

Boxed cereal wasn't meant to be sweet, nor made of refined wheat. At the end of the nineteenth century, in an effort to replicate the making of granola (known as a food contributing to good health) a man by the name of John Harvey Kellogg experimented with wheat by boiling it, rolling it into thin flakes, then baking it. He soon found he had the perfect, no-cooking-needed breakfast cereal on his hands, a food that could be packaged and sold by the box.

But it wouldn't be until a half century later that cold boxed cereal would be swimming in sugar, partly in an effort to lure kids into eating cereal (think Frosted Flakes, Froot Loops, and Cocoa Puffs), and made in a way that transformed it from a simply made, wholesome food to a heavily processed, sweet one. Cereal out of a box, the most popular breakfast choice in America, has become the most adulterated breakfast food in history.

Before there was boxed cereal, there was hot cereal, the kind of cereal people had been eating for millennia, what we refer to now as porridge. It usually consisted of a whole cereal grain (wheat, millet, rye, oats, rice, etc.) slow-cooked with water.

Modifications to this original, WAMP cereal can be found all over the world throughout the course of history and today. The Chinese call their rice version *congee*; the Russians call a buckwheat variety *kasha*; the Iranians have a wheat version they call *halim*; and the South Indians enjoy one called *upma*, a fried semolina (wheat) porridge made with butter, onions, mustard seeds, and a variety of fresh vegetables.

A Tall Latte and a Doughnut

The idea of *needing* to pair our morning coffee with something sweet has everything to do with why our breakfast needs a reboot. It wasn't until nearly a decade after Starbucks first opened its doors in 1971 that the chain added pastries and banana breads, now described as "breakfast snacks," to its menu. Before that, it was simply a coffeehouse, serving only coffee. These days, in a fight to get a bigger share of our valuable breakfast dollars, restaurant chains are cleverly packaging the concept of coffee plus a floury, sweet treat into combo meals, whereby the purchase of a latte gets you a piece of coffee cake for a sweet (no pun intended) price.

The bottom line is that our modern-day breakfast lineup has veered way off-course from its origins, origins that were based on WAMP eating. Today's breakfast has been strategically concocted to limit you and to seduce your taste buds in all the wrong ways.

Ready for a Better Breakfast?

It's time to open our hearts, minds, and kitchens to a new and improved breakfast, one that doesn't mean just cereal, toast, pancakes, and bagels.

Let's start by taking a tour around the world to see how other cultures start their day. Although many countries do indeed have their own versions of sweet, flour-based items for breakfast, these foods aren't as heavily processed. For instance, in some countries you're likely to find a flatbread or fried bread-like item, but the bread will likely be made with a less refined flour (and not just wheat flour).

For example, in Burma breakfast might include a buttered flatbread, soup, rice or noodles, and peas. If you had a seat at a restaurant in Tokyo or at many fine hotels in America, you'd come across the famous Japanese breakfast: broiled fish; steamed rice; miso soup made with tofu, wakame (a type of seaweed), and scallions; natto (fermented

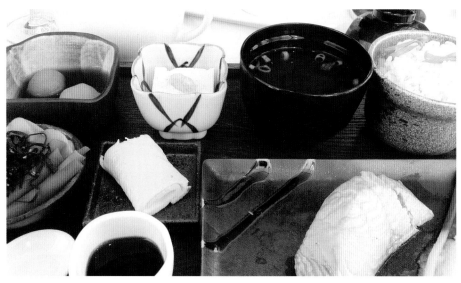

A classic Japanese breakfast

soy beans); a small rolled omelet called *tamagoyaki* with grated daikon radish; and a small dish of pickled vegetables. To drink? No latte or espresso, only some wonderfully aromatic jasmine green tea.

In Malaysia, you might get a hot bowl called *mee* that consists of noodles mixed with eggs, vegetables, and spices. In Jordan, tea, hummus, and falafels. In Costa Rica, black beans, rice, sour cream, salsa, and corn tortillas are staples. On a recent trip to the Caribbean, I stayed at an Asian hotel chain and received a breakfast of my dreams: a hot bowl of chicken-and-rice soup seasoned with spices and lemongrass. It was divine.

Another huge distinction between the average American breakfast and those we see in other countries is the use of more vegetable proteins as opposed to animal proteins. Less sausage and bacon drowning in oil, and more beans, lentils, and high-protein whole grains. Who says we can't eat chickpea hummus, quinoa, or black beans in the *morning*?

Global breakfasts show us that we need more diversity and more nourishing, WAMP ingredients in our morning meal. People around the world eat a plethora of ingredients, from fish and lentils to spices and rice. A variety of ingredients is key because that's where better flavor comes from. Instead of choosing sweet, we need to tap into sour, savory, salty, and even spicy in the morning!

Instead of sticking to wheat flour for breakfast, discover brown rice, polenta, and other whole grains. Instead of a boring fruit cup, indulge in a dish that includes greens. Who says we can't enjoy cilantro in the morning? Or radishes, or quinoa, or arugula, or basil? Bring on the vegetables and herbs! Whether pickled, steamed, or raw, vegetables are key to many breakfasts across the planet. Sure, we're used to potatoes and maybe some onions, bell peppers, and tomatoes, but that's that the extent of it. Who says we can't broaden our horizons? Who says our breakfast can't look more like our more nutrient-dense lunch, or even our dinner? They don't have to. You are in charge!

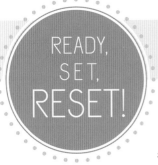

I've read countless methods for improving one's life, such as how to mediate, how to be effective at time management, how to be a great public speaker. But only after I put these tools into practice could I learn and grow. That's what this Reset chapter is all about. In order to make revolutionary, long-term, healthy shifts to the way we eat our breakfast, we need to experience the change first. It's not enough just to read about it. We need to do it.

I'm here to help you make and taste four different, delectable breakfast recipes that are guaranteed to make you want to change up your breakfast routine. You will discover how the use of fresh, whole, and diverse ingredients can redefine your AM yum!

Instructions

Here's how we will do it: Over the next three days, you will refrain from any and all breakfast food that's not WAMP. This means no sugary cereals, bagels, or scones.

You will also avoid drinking anything overly sweet for breakfast. This means no bottled Frappuccinos or sweetened drinks like vanilla lattes or mochas. Unsweetened coffee, espresso drinks, and teas are ideal. Sweeten them as little as you can.

In exchange, you will make the wildly flavorful recipes below in the comfort of your own kitchen. These recipes are short and easy. For example, the Quinoa Coconut Cereal is meant as a substitute for processed, boxed cereal. The Smoked Salmon Breakfast Pita is an alternative to various breakfast sandwiches made with processed meats and breads. The Tofu Curry Scramble shows off vegetables, vegetarian protein, and introduces your palette to savory, umami, and spicy in the morning—flavors that will awaken your senses and taste buds! As a fourth recipe option, I've included the Banana-Cinnamon Rice Cereal from the Wheat Reset chapter.

Go ahead and choose your three favorites, one for each of the three days. Or, to make things even easier, pick one recipe and repeat it. I realize that for many of you, cooking in the morning, even if it's fast is still a tall order. But remember, it's only three days!

It's not easy to change a ritual that has been so engrained in our lives and culture. Please be patient. Keep your mind and heart open. You will be rewarded for the time and energy you're about to invest!

TIPS & TOOLS for EACH DAY

Day One

Good morning! Today you will start reprogramming the way you enjoy breakfast for life. If you've been eating the same brand of boxed cereal in the same bowl, seated in the same chair, for years on end, this isn't going to be the easiest of transitions. But hold on. What you're about to eat will make up for it.

Today you might want to try the Smoked Salmon Breakfast Pita because it's easy to make, quick, very satisfying, and more conventional than the other recipes. When making this recipe, make sure you're using 100 percent whole-wheat pita bread. When you take the first bite and taste the sweet freshness of the basil, the richness of the salmon, the creaminess of the avocado, and the spiciness of Tabasco sauce, you'll find it tantalizing!

With this recipe, consider how veggie proteins and fats like avocado can be just as

WAMP Breakfast	Refined Sugars	Refined Wheat Flour	WAMP Grains	WAMP Fruits & Veggies	WAMP Protein
Quinoa-Coconut Cereal	none	none	√	√	√
Smoked Salmon Breakfast Pita	none	none	√	√	√
Tofu-Curry Scramble	none	none	√	√	√
Banana-Cinnamon Rice Cereal	none	none	√	√	√

filling as animal proteins. Also think about how little we eat fish in the morning, whereas fish is considered a foundational ingredient in many breakfasts around the world.

If you don't have time to eat your breakfast after you make it, this particular recipe does well as a to-go meal. Just wrap it up in plastic wrap or aluminum foil, and you're ready to head to work.

Tonight, as a time-saver, consider making the quinoa now if you're interested in trying the Quinoa Coconut Cereal tomorrow. You will save yourself a good fifteen minutes in the morning. Quinoa is very easy. After it's done cooking, just let it cool, place it in a storage container, and put it in the fridge.

Day Two

You're almost halfway there! It's time for the quinoa cereal. This recipe will make you rethink cold, boxed breakfast cereal! If you made the quinoa last night, pull it from the fridge and heat it with the milk of your choice in the microwave if you want to enjoy this recipe hot. Otherwise, just follow the recipe instructions.

I find this cereal to be a game-changer because (1) I've never had a client or friend tell me it wasn't over-the-top delicious, (2) it's the perfect way to showcase the tastiness of whole grains as opposed to refined cereals and bagels, and (3) it allows us to get the sweetness we're after without processed sugar.

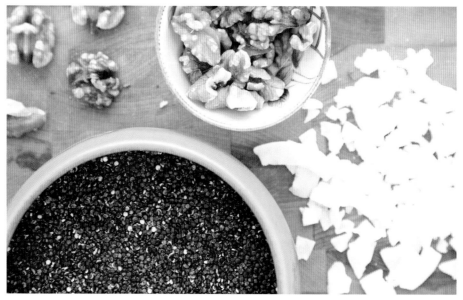

Simple and WAMP: red quinoa, walnuts, and coconut flakes

Don't be put off by the coconut flakes if you've never tasted them before or haven't used them in this way. Dry coconut meat—which is what these flakes are—has an exotic flavor, and combined with the raisins it yields the perfect WAMP sweetness. What makes this dish so great is this sweetness combined with the nutty crunchiness of the quinoa. The combination is extraordinary.

Quinoa is rich in protein, so every bite is satisfying and won't leave you craving more, as sugar-laden, boxed cereals do. If you want to double the recipe, it's easy to store an extra serving for tomorrow or for another family member.

As you continue your day, take a minute or two to look at the breakfast offerings that routinely surround you. What do they offer at your office pantry or cafeteria in the morning? What do your colleagues or friends routinely eat? What do fast-food chains or delis serve, and how does the flavor compare with what you just ate?

Day Three

Good for you, you're almost done! This morning, it's time to try one of the final two recipes. Both help to solidify the concepts of this Reset in different ways. The Tofu

Scramble makes veggie protein king for breakfast, something that traditional American breakfasts don't do, and it's jam-packed with potent flavor. Instead of the conventional greasy animal proteins that come standard in American breakfasts—sausages, ham, and bacon—notice how vegetarian proteins (tofu, beans, etc.) can satisfy us in similar ways. The Banana-Cinnamon Rice Cereal teaches us something similar to what we learned from the Quinoa Coconut Cereal: that whole grains and WAMP sweetness trump refined flour and refined sugar any day. Brown rice is one of the easiest and best substitutes for refined wheat flour, and bananas and cinnamon are far more nutritious and flavorful than table sugar.

After the Reset

Congratulations on finishing your Reset! You are now freed from the notion that break-fast *must* mean cereal, toast, and pancakes. This Reset has given you the opportunity to enjoy not only a more delicious breakfast, but a healthier one. Your taste buds have had a short respite from the manipulative and sabotaging traits of processed breakfast foods.

Consider yourself renewed and empowered. With your new knowledge and skill set, you now know that quinoa (and the entire spectrum of whole grains, such as brown rice and oats) can be substituted for all white breads and baked goods: muffins, scones, bagels, croissants, etc.

You now have the confidence to navigate breakfast in any situation—whether at a morning meeting, an all-day conference, or the airport. When all you see in front of you is a sea of pastries, bagels, and sugar-coated scones, you won't be fooled. You'll look instead for fruit, eggs, unsweetened oatmeal, or other WAMP alternatives. Or you might have packed your breakfast ahead of time! You'll be more creative when seeking breakfast foods and more open to enjoying a broader range of flavors.

Here is some additional guidance to help you on your way:

- There are a variety of whole grains you can eat to substitute for wheat, such as brown rice, quinoa, and whole oats. They're easy to find and make, especially if you have a rice cooker. Just pop them in at night and presto, they're done for you in the morning. I recommend investing in a rice cooker by Zojirushi.

- If you need sweetness in the morning, you can make many modifications to the quinoa cereal recipe. WAMP sweetness can come not only from raisins and coconuts, but also from cinnamon, dates, pears (and many other fruits), honey, and maple syrup. Feel free to experiment. Instead of quinoa, try brown rice. My favorite easy breakfast is cooked brown rice mashed up with a ripe banana, half an avocado, and a dash or two of ground cinnamon—fast and delicious!

- Start to investigate other breakfast products and brands, especially cereal brands that are more WAMP and less processed. Look for those that are unsweetened. Scan the ingredient list for refined sugars (see the Sugar Reset chapter for a discussion and list of processed sweeteners). My two favorite cereals are Food for Life's Ezekiel and Familia Swiss Muesli ("No Added Sugar" version). Check your local natural foods or health food store for both.

- Don't be afraid to eat veggies and fish in the morning. Think about smoked salmon and beans more often, as well as vegetable leftovers from last night's dinner. Since dinners—especially WAMP dinners—tend to be more nutrient dense than breakfasts, why not nourish yourself with PM food in the AM?

- Follow the 80/20 Rule. If you find you're eating scones, French toast, or waffles at a beautiful outdoor Sunday brunch with your family, no need to worry. If you can eat WAMP breakfasts 80 percent of the time, don't feel guilty about the other 20 percent.

- Be creative and use whatever is in your refrigerator. Breakfast needs to be fast and impromptu for most of us. Sometimes throwing together some scrambled eggs with fresh herbs, greens, tomatoes, pesto, and salt and pepper is just the ticket. As long as your food is WAMP, you're golden.

- In the end, remember this: Conventional breakfast has us fooled. If you see the same options everywhere you turn, don't break under the peer pressure. Stand your ground and feel confident in taking a different route. Your friends will soon be taking your lead!

YOUR BREAKFAST RESET GROCERY LIST

- ☐ 1 c quinoa, rinsed and drained (or about 3 c cooked quinoa)
- ☐ Sea salt
- ☐ 1/2 c chopped walnuts
- ☐ 1/2 c dried unsweetened coconut flakes
- ☐ Unsweetened almond milk, cow's milk, or other unsweetened nut milk
- ☐ 1/2 c raisins
- ☐ Honey (optional)
- ☐ Whole-wheat pita
- ☐ Pasture butter, or organic expeller-pressed canola oil or olive oil
- ☐ 1 organic egg
- ☐ 1 package smoked wild salmon
- ☐ 1 lemon
- ☐ 1 avocado
- ☐ 1 ripe organic or heirloom tomato
- ☐ 1 bunch fresh basil

- ☐ Tabasco sauce
- ☐ Balsamic vinegar
- ☐ Extra-virgin olive oil
- ☐ 1 bulb garlic
- ☐ 1 yellow or red onion
- ☐ 1 red bell pepper
- ☐ 6 oz mushrooms
- ☐ 4 c baby spinach
- ☐ 14 oz firm tofu
- ☐ Bragg Liquid Aminos (or low-sodium soy sauce)
- ☐ Pimenton or smoked paprika (optional)
- ☐ Ground cumin
- ☐ Curry powder
- ☐ Worcestershire sauce
- ☐ Ground black pepper
- ☐ Cilantro (optional)

Quinoa Coconut Cereal

This recipe is the perfect example of how delicious WAMP foods can be! Coconut flakes, raisins, and honey are the perfect WAMP sweeteners, while quinoa adds nuttiness, crunch, and texture to wow our senses.

SERVES: 4
TOTAL TIME: 20 MINUTES

INGREDIENTS

- 1 1/2 c quinoa, rinsed and drained (or about 3 c cooked quinoa)
- 1/4 tsp sea salt
- 2 1/4 c filtered water
- 1/2 c chopped walnuts
- 1/2 c dried unsweetened coconut flakes
- 2 c unsweetened almond milk, cow's milk, or other nut milk
- 1/2 c raisins
- Raw honey to taste (optional)

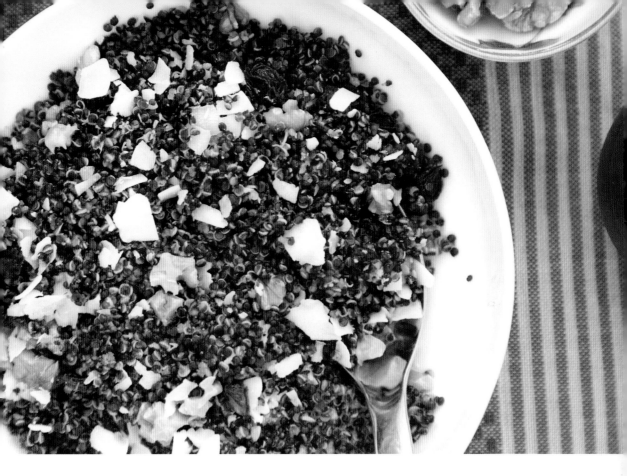

PROCEDURE

1. Place quinoa in a saucepan over medium heat. Stir a minute or two, slighting toasting the quinoa. Then add salt, water, cover and bring to a boil. Reduce heat to a simmer and cook, covered, for 15 minutes, or until the quinoa seed has unfurled (the spiral-like germ emerges) and all the water has been absorbed. Turn off the heat and allow it to sit, covered to steam a few more minutes.

2. Place quinoa in large serving bowl. Add the remaining ingredients and stir to combine. Divide among cereal bowls and add honey on top if desired.

Smoked Salmon Breakfast Pita

This pita sandwich trumps any breakfast sandwich you'd get from the deli. It shows off the beautiful flavors and aromas that come from using fresh, WAMP ingredients like basil, lemon, and avocado. Protein and healthy fat from the avocado make this meal nourishing and energizing.

SERVES: 1
TOTAL TIME: 15 MINUTES

INGREDIENTS

- 1/2 whole wheat flour pita
- 1/2 tsp pasture butter, or organic expeller-pressed canola oil
- 1 organic egg
- Sea salt and fresh ground pepper to taste
- 2 x 4-inch piece smoked wild sockeye salmon
- 1/2 lemon
- 1/4–1/2 avocado, sliced into 1/4-inch pieces
- 1–2 slices ripe organic or heirloom tomato (sliced crosswise into 1/4-inch thick piece, then halved
- 3–5 fresh basil leaves
- Tabasco sauce
- Balsamic vinegar

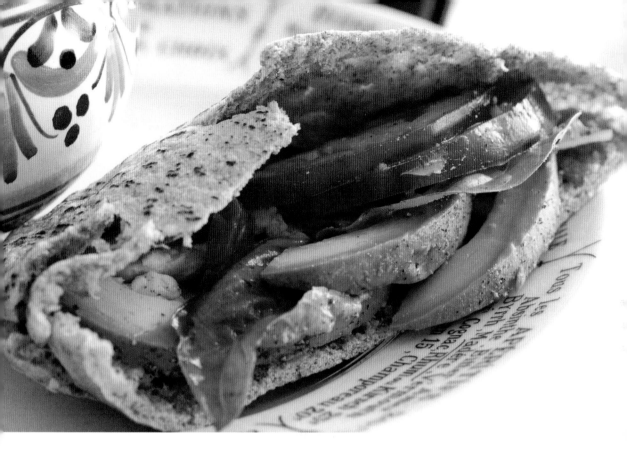

PROCEDURE

1. Toast pita in toaster oven or toaster. Remove and let sit.

2. Heat the butter or oil in a small frying pan over low heat. When the pan becomes coated, add the egg and scramble over medium-low heat. Remove the egg and season it with salt and pepper.

3. Start filling your pita. Add the eggs and salmon first, dressing the salmon with a few squeezes of lemon. Follow with the avocado, tomato, and basil. Season again with salt, pepper, Tabasco, and balsamic to taste. Enjoy immediately or wrap and pack for the office.

Notes:

• Instead of scrambling eggs, opt for a hard-boiled egg. You can cook your hard-boiled egg the night before to make this recipe even faster.

• If you don't have basil on hand, use baby arugula or baby spinach. Mix and match to your taste.

Tofu Curry Scramble

This recipe redefines breakfast flavor! It's all about proportions and seasoning so if you enjoy more veggies, add more and if the seasoning is not quite right, experiment with the amount of Worcestershire sauce, Liquid Aminos, and curry powder.

 SERVES: 4
TOTAL TIME: 15 MINUTES

INGREDIENTS

- 2 tbsp, plus 2 tsp extra-virgin olive oil
- 5 garlic cloves, finely minced
- 1 c red or yellow onion, small dice
- 1 c red bell pepper, small dice
- 2 c chopped mushrooms
- 4 c baby spinach, packed
- 14 oz firm tofu
- 4 tsp Braggs Liquid Aminos (or low sodium soy sauce)
- 1/2 tsp pimenton or smoked paprika (optional)
- 1/2 tsp ground cumin
- 2 tsp curry powder
- 4 tsp Worcestershire sauce
- 1/4 tsp fresh ground black pepper
- chopped cilantro (for garnish, optional)

Notes:

• Bragg Liquid Aminos is a low-sodium substitute for soy sauce. You can find it at most grocery stores.

• If you need a little more spiciness, try adding Tabasco sauce or minced green chilies.

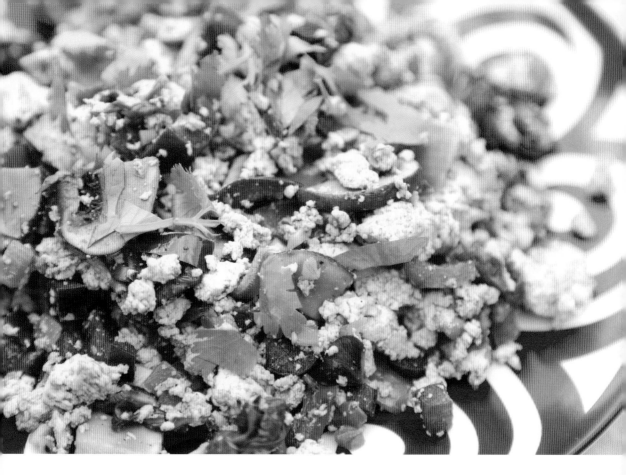

PROCEDURE

1. Place a frying pan over high heat and add 5 teaspoons oil. When it is hot, add the onions and garlic. Sauté until the onions begin to caramelize. Be careful not to burn the garlic.

2. Add peppers and mushrooms and sauté for another few minutes. Then add spinach and continue to sauté until the spinach is entirely wilted.

3. Remove vegetables and set aside.

4. In the same pan, warm the remaining oil over medium heat. When hot, crumble tofu into the pan using your fingers. Fry the tofu for a few minutes.

5. Add the vegetables back into the pan with the tofu and mix to incorporate. Turn heat to low and add all the remaining seasonings. Cook for another minute.

6. Plate, garnish with cilantro, and enjoy.

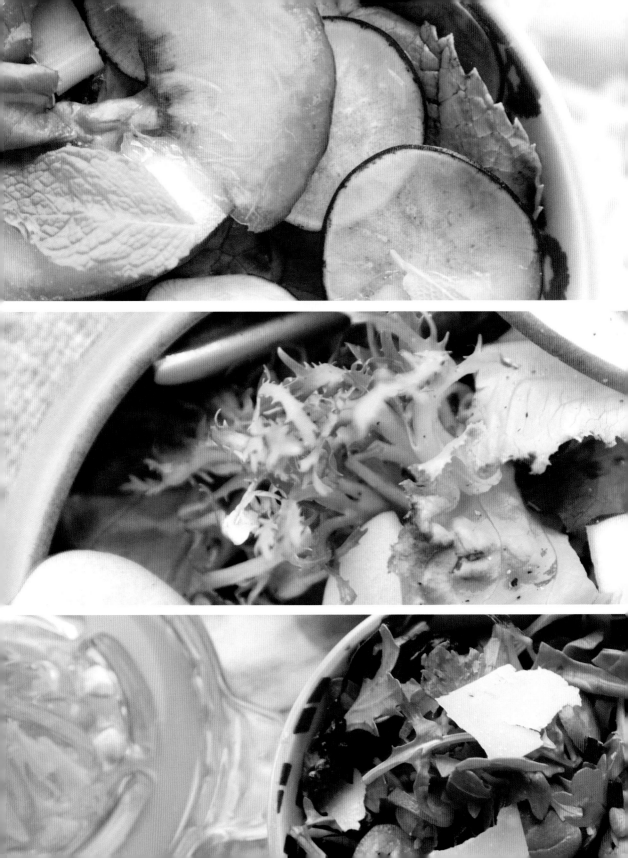

CHANGE

Salad
RESET

When I was growing up in the 1980s, my parents would take my brother and me to Ponderosa Steakhouse for a well-priced, all-you-can-eat salad bar on the weekends. I'd head straight to the bar, plate in hand, and load up on carrots, cucumbers, peas, lettuce, diced peppers, and cooked chickpeas. Next came my favorite part, the accompaniments: mountains of seasoned croutons, grated cheese, and then the pièce de résistance, a few generous—very generous—ladles of Catalina dressing. Delish!

I loved these jaunts to Ponderosa, but it wouldn't be until nearly two decades later that I realized exactly *why*. It wasn't for the vegetables. I liked getting my all-you-can-eat salad specifically because of the fixings I dumped over the top—the perfect meld of food-science-engineered sweet, fatty, and salty. To be honest, the flavor of the dressing itself was so overwhelming that I can't remember the taste of much else. My taste buds didn't care about the subtle and unique flavors inherent in the greens and veggies; instead, they were fixated on the processed flavors of the shredded cheese, dressing, and greasy croutons.

News flash: That Ponderosa salad I craved so much as a kid *wasn't really salad*. And neither are those tossed "garden salads" encased in plastic to-go containers that populate refrigerated sections of countless cafés, delis, and lunchrooms across the country.

These types of salads aren't any more authentic than canned Chef Boyardee is real Italian pasta.

The salads that surround us today are nowhere near what the originals looked like hundreds of years ago. Today's salads have been compromised. They've lost their true identity, and, as a result, their flavor and health benefits. The best tasting salads in our history were made from the simplest, freshest, ripest, whole ingredients, with very few "fixings."

The makers of today's salads have committed a culinary crime. Most salads aren't made in a way that makes them look or taste good. The flawed mainstream understanding of what *must* comprise a salad—iceberg lettuce, raw mushrooms, diced onions, and the like—has left much to be desired. This is a shame because real salads are, by nature, some of the most elegant, glorious, and delectable culinary creations in the world.

> In this Reset, we will overhaul this dish so much that instead of feeling unexcited by its taste, or overly reliant on processed dressings, you'll find yourself relishing simple salads!

The standardization and blandness forces us to pile on the bacon bits, croutons, hunks of cheese, and creamy dressings—all resulting in a salad that has much more in common with processed food than it does with WAMP food.

If there's one thing that's corrupted salad the most, it's all that bottled "fat-free ranch" and "creamy French" that occupy miles of grocery-store shelf space, compliments of the food-processing industry. Not only do they manipulate our cravings but they also drown out the flavors of the veggies underneath, preventing us from enjoying salad the way we should be. Authentic salad dressings were the epitome of wholesomeness and minimalism. No sugar was added, no artificial flavorings, no ingredient labels—just olive oil and vinegars.

In this Reset, we will reverse course and completely change the way we define and enjoy salads. We will overhaul this dish so much that instead of feeling unexcited by its taste, or overly reliant on processed dressings and other such accompaniments, you'll find yourself relishing simple salads and even wanting to make them from scratch day after day! In the next seventy-two-hours, you'll discover how true salads made with WAMP ingredients are the best examples of delicious *and* healthy eating.

Salad's Salad Days: What You Need to Know About Salad

The history of salad can give us many clues as to why the modern incarnation falls short. It begins with vegetables, which have been playing a role in the human diet since the Bronze Age, when olives and grapes—the yin and yang of French vinaigrettes—were discovered, somewhere between 4000 and 3000 BC. Radishes, carrots, and spinach were also popular foods about a thousand years ago.

The Greeks and Romans should be credited with the invention of the WAMP salad. The Greeks loved lettuce and considered it the "best of all salad plants." It was believed to be both an aphrodisiac and a sleep aid. As the story goes, Venus slept on a bed of lettuce to forget her lost Adonis. In love with greens, Greeks were the first to "dress" raw veggies with a combination of oil, vinegar, and brine (a solution of salt in water), which interestingly generated the etymology of the dish: *Sal*—Latin for "salt"—best described the salty flavor of this ancient way of seasoning. Hence salad got its name from the character of the liquids it was coated in—what we now refer to as "dressing." It wasn't until the 1400s, however, that versions of the word "salad" first began appearing in languages. The dish came to be referred to as *zelade* in fifteenth-century Italy and, soon after, *salade* in French.

The French were so fond of eating vegetables that they built lavish gardens for their royalty. The Potager du Roi, or Kitchen Garden of the King, was constructed for Louis XIV in 1678 near his Palace of Versailles, enabling his staff to conduct "careful selection of the perfectly ripened produce" and indulge in the freshest of salads. The French king apparently had a weakness for the dish. It's been said he ate a prodigious quantity of salad year-round because it was refreshing, aided in digestion, and promoted good sleep and appetite.

Salad making was considered a skill. Royalty and the upper class often called on the finest salad makers to prepare the most tempting dressings and the most delicious combination of greens. Salad was indeed a gourmet dish, respected and enjoyed for its tempting flavors, textures, and nourishment.

Salad Bars and Other Modern Inventions

Fast-forward to the twentieth century, when salads began a grand transformation, taking on an entirely new roster of names and conventions, all of American design. In 1924, an immigrant restaurateur by the name of Caesar Cardini developed the Caesar salad prepared primarily with romaine lettuce, Parmesan cheese, croutons, and Worcestershire sauce. The same decade brought us the bacon-, egg-, and chicken-heavy Cobb salad. Thousand Island dressing was also a twentieth-century American invention.

One of the biggest modifications to salad came in the 1960s when "salad bars," like the ones I frequented as a child, began springing up across countless delis, restaurant chains, and office cafeterias, the genius of restaurateur and Colorado native Norman Brinker. With this innovation, salads lost their beauty, flavor, variety, and authenticity. Although supposedly fresh, ingredients at salad bars sat around in bins, withering for hours, victims of oxidation. And instead of offering people the freedom to choose ingredients that were in season and ripe (the most flavorful), these salad bars now held all the power, some even providing items from cans (like corn and peas). Instead of giving people the option of making simple, healthful dressings with their own two hands, salad bars offered mega-sized, sugar-filled, processed dressings that could be flipped upside down and dredged over the dish. And let's not forget the add-ons. Things like oily croutons, processed meats, and other fixings became part and parcel of salad bars.

From Craving to Coaxing

Over the last century, we've taken salads from WAMP to processed. They've become dishes that we endure rather than savor, tolerate rather than celebrate. We've transformed them from grandiose, mouthwatering plates of nourishment to stale, flavorless, run-of-the-mill side dishes we feel coaxed into eating in order to stay "healthy" and get "skinny." Instead of craving salads, we now associate them with restraint, obligation, and sacrifice.

Three factors are mainly to blame: processed dressings, inferior ingredients, and a loss of creativity.

All Dressed Up

Salad dressings were meant to be simple. The Greeks used just vinegar, olive oil, and brine. As dressings evolved through the centuries, eggs were added, and in some countries yogurt and sour cream also became core ingredients—the basis for creamy dressings.

Dressings changed for the worse in the 1980s when food scientists figured out how to create artificial flavors to mimic perishable ingredients like buttermilk and eggs—ingredients that otherwise required refrigeration. Dressings suddenly became shelf stable and could be bottled in glass or plastic, slapped with an expiry date, and stored for months—the processed salad industry had arrived.

Today's store bought dressings contain much more than just a few WAMP ingredients. The salt, sugar, fat, and additive-infused dressings we use today wreak havoc on our taste buds while drowning out healthy flavor. Xantham gum, potassium sorbate and "natural flavoring" are standard ingredients in processed, store-bought dressings.

The tragedy here is that salad dressings may well be the easiest condiment to make in our kitchens. Problem is, most of us don't know how.

Common Ingredients in Store-Bought Dressings

- Sorbic acid
- Xantham gum
- Soybean oil
- Natural flavor
- Sugar

- Sodium benzoate
- Caramel color
- Annatto extract (color)
- Corn syrup
- Soybean oil

- Maltodextrin
- Expeller-pressed vegetable oil
- Phosphoric acid
- Potassium sorbate
- Calcium disodium EDTA

> ### Ingredient Lists Lie
>
> Even though you may see a bottled salad dressing ingredient list that includes "tomato," "garlic," "black pepper," and other WAMP ingredients, this doesn't mean the dressing isn't processed. The tomatoes are certainly not fresh, nor is the garlic. Keep in mind that to ensure dressings are shelf-stable, a lot of processing must be involved—they're not WAMP.

Salad's Inferiority Is Complex

Yet even if we got the dressing right, today's salad is still incredibly lacking because we're not using the right base ingredients. In most instances, the vegetables on our salad plates were harvested before their prime and shipped to us from hundreds of miles away. By the time the romaine, carrots, corn, and tomatoes reach our forks, they've been wasting away in transit, deadened by weeks in a can, or limp from the oxidation that occurs from sitting in a large tub at your neighborhood grocery-store salad bar. Average grocery-store produce is rarely tasty, but since that's where we usually buy our food, we don't know any better.

We expect produce to be dull and bland. We don't question the crispness from a bite of a spinach leaf, the degree of crunch from a stick of celery, or the level of sweetness from a tomato—all clues that signal superior quality. We've settled.

King Louis XIV understood this perfectly when he ordered the creation of a kitchen garden on the palace grounds to ensure he had the freshest produce to make the best-tasting salads. Granted, we all can't have backyard gardens, but the understanding that the best flavor comes from quality and freshness is free.

Mix It Up

Another contributor to the downfall of salad: We've stopped requiring a mélange of flavors, textures, colors, and aromas. There's no good reason to settle for the classic airplane salad of iceberg lettuce, julienned stale carrots, and a scant dropping of cherry tomatoes. That's *not* a salad; that's rabbit food!

Dressing Factoids

Four of the top five salad dressings in America—Thousand Island, Ranch, Caesar, and American-style Italian—are twentieth-century commercial creations. Invented in 1952, the original recipe for ranch dressing was eventually bought by the Clorox company, the same company that makes Pine-Sol and Liquid Plumr.

Sticking with the same monotonous ticker tape of ingredients every time won't make salads worth craving. The flavor potential of salads hugely depends on mixing and matching fresh herbs, fruits, a variety of greens, and unique combinations of vegetables in order to heighten tastes such as savory, bitter, sweet, and umami—tastes that if combined together in balanced ways are guaranteed to please the human palate.

Basil, mint, thyme, grapefruit, endive, butter lettuce, scallions, and red onions can all be mixed and matched in ways that produce wildly flavorful combinations that arouse, seduce, and enliven. How about some raspberries, mint, and orange zest? Didn't think these could be salad ingredients? They can be! Even some flower petals, like nasturtium, are edible and make beautiful, colorful salad toppers.

Salad Skills

I grant you that vegetables can be intimidating to prepare. Even if we skip the grocery store and buy glorious, fresh, WAMP produce at a farmers' market, who knows what to do with a big bunch of arugula with the soil still clinging to its roots? Or, without a recipe, how to cook the beets that we bought because we know that somehow they "must be good for us"?

There's something about produce that puts up red flags. We think it's too labor-intensive to rinse, dry, peel, chop, and slice; too taxing to clean up the mess. So, we end up not eating what we buy and sending it to the trash (or the green bin) despite our good intentions. Instead, we fill up on easy-to-grab, no-cooking-involved foods like processed bread, cheese, cereal, pasta, and yogurt. No wonder we Americans barely make our recommended fruit- and vegetable-consumption quotas.

The Art of Salad

Salad-making is like art. It stimulates the senses, gives you freedom to unleash your creativity, and enlivens you. The best salads radiate myriad colors, from dark purple to mustard yellow, mint green to pomegranate red. Combining distinctive flavors from fruits, vegetables, greens, and herbs light up our taste buds with bursts of pungent, tangy, tart, and sweet. Plant foods are beautiful little creatures; they are Mother Nature's Picassos, Miros, and Monets. Just looking at them can inspire, calm, and uplift. Eating them makes us feel fresh, alive, and vital. Good salads are easily within our reach; we just need the right skills to unlock their potential and our inner artist.

Let me be the first to tell you, though, that salad-making is nothing more than a simple, lost skill that can be resurrected easily and in one trip to the kitchen. Preparing salads can be one of the most satisfying ways to "cook" that you could ever imagine. Once we realize how easy it is to do, the fear of peeling, chopping, and time drain will be eliminated. Shopping won't go to waste. And your motivation to eat what you've created will skyrocket. That's what you'll be learning soon in this Reset.

It won't be difficult, I promise. About a year ago I was invited to be the guest market chef at a Saturday farmers' market in downtown San Francisco. There was no protocol as to what recipes we could showcase there, with one exception: The ingredients had to be seasonal and available for purchase that day, at the market.

After considering a tofu, a tempeh, and even a chicken dish, I finally decided to make something much more simple—laughably simple almost! After all, I had a six-month-old baby to look after, and little time for prep work, so I chose a basil and orange salad with a miso dressing. It required no cooking, just a blender and a few ingredients for the dressing, and minimal chopping.

It was one of the easiest recipes I'd ever taught. It also turned out to be one of the biggest hits. The audience loved the unique umami flavor of the dressing, and found that it complemented the bitterness of the greens and the sweetness of the citrus brilliantly. One woman exclaimed that she couldn't believe there was no oil in the dressing. (There

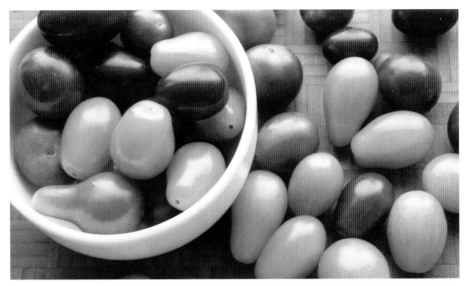

Cherry tomatoes: colorful, nourishing, and sweet

wasn't.) The crowd left my demonstration with a whole new perspective on salad, not to mention a new sense of empowerment, confident they could recreate the dish in their own kitchens.

I went home thinking that salads have to be some of the most gratifying dishes on Earth. They're insanely simple to make from scratch, uniquely flavorful, and tremendously healthy. One of the most detrimental lies in our modern eating culture is that we can't make the tastiest, most delicious salads and dressings *on our own*. Salads don't require anything more than a knife, bowl, whisk, and cutting board! That we need some five-star chef to make them appetizing is beyond wrong.

Under no circumstances does a salad have to be a "sacrificial dish"—a food appropriate only to the dieter or the strong-willed. There should be only one requirement when eating a salad: You love it.

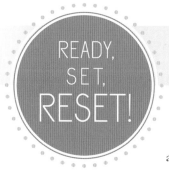

READY,
SET,
RESET!

Now that you know how off-kilter our relationship with salads is, it's time for a Reset. We will throw on our aprons and get our knives and cutting boards out. We will erase any and all preconceived notions of "salad" and open our minds and palettes to something new. We will put flavor first because that's what 3DR is all about: falling in love with nutritious *and delicious* food!

Over the next three days, you will have the chance to cook and enjoy three unconventional salad recipes. Experiencing these three dishes will underscore four important factors in effectively resetting salad.

First, in order for us to enjoy salad the right way, we need to make sure all the ingredients we use are WAMP—or better yet, Super WAMP. Most vegetables, greens, and fruits come to us in whole-food form, yet we must keep freshness and ripeness in mind. Freshness and ripeness are paramount for one reason and one reason alone: They determine flavor. For most plant matter, the shorter the time between harvest and your first bite, the more exquisite the flavor. As for ripeness, try tasting a tomato harvested before its peak vs. one that's picked at the perfect time. The tomato picked at the right time will taste a million times better.

To capitalize on flavor, do your best to buy your produce from farmers' markets, where you get food directly from a farmer in your area (which decreases transit time). This produce is also both in season and likely harvested at the right time.

Second, in enjoying these three salads, you will break free from the idea that salads have to look a certain way or follow the status quo. You'll learn that salad-making is free-form, and no ingredient is off limits. By getting intimate with a variety of unique ingredients, you'll realize that no two vegetables taste alike. No two herbs. No two fruits. Arugula is bitter, chard more mild. Mint is aromatic with a cooling aftertaste. Rosemary is more astringent. Lettuce is tender and refreshing. And carrots are sweet and slightly nutty. Any item you put in your salad has its own distinct character. Some salads combine

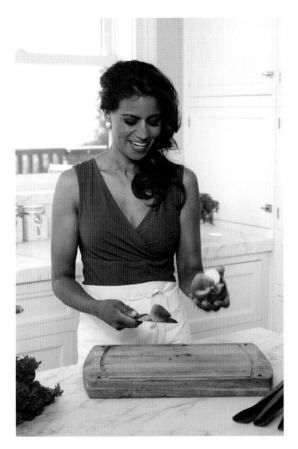

pomegranates with pineapple, chili flakes, and cumin, while the Japanese utilize mizuna greens, daikon radish, miso, ginger, and sesame seeds. In other words, there is no *right way* to make a salad. So the more you use variety to your advantage, the more you can manipulate, mix, match, and maximize flavor.

Third, this seventy-two-hour experience will help you understand the power behind balancing flavors. Sure, Super WAMP carrots taste great on their own as they're per-fectly sweet, but alongside a spicy arugula leaf, the taste experience goes up a notch. That's how our palates work—they revel in yin and yang. As touched upon early in this book, the interaction of complex flavors is what continually surprises our taste buds. That's part of the art of cooking. So including a bitter vegetable like radicchio that's balanced on the other end with something sweet, like orange segments or pears, will make our taste buds happier than eating either ingredient alone. It's this synergy that ultimately makes our mouths water. You'll see!

Last but definitely not least, this Reset will help you understand the true role of dressings in salad. You'll realize that dressings are merely meant to enhance the ingredients they dress, not dominate them. Think of it as putting on a beautiful ball gown or tuxedo for an extravagant affair. You choose such a garment carefully so it will help you show off your body's features and your beauty rather than hiding your best attributes. That's the role of dressings. The best-tasting dressings can be made in your kitchen with just a bowl and a whisk, or even in a jar with a tight lid. And just as with the salad itself, the flavor

Oil and Vinegar

We all know that oil and vinegar don't mix. Put them in a jar and have a robot shake it for hours and you'll still never see them combine. That's because their chemical makeup won't allow for it, and why dressings usually contain emulsifiers—ingredients that help bring two otherwise unblendable liquids together. Some of the most common emulsifers are egg yolks, mustard, or garlic, which, when added to vinegar and oil, allow these two polarizing substances to hold together by affixing themselves to both. In other words, they act as the bridge.

The most flavorful salad dressings always contain an emulsifer. To achieve the most technically sound emulsification, whisk the vinegar, emulsifier, and all ingredients, except the oil, first. Then, while still whisking, add the oil in a slow and steady stream.

of a dressing can be maximized by using a variety of ingredients. Citrus juices, herbs, soy sauce, raspberries, and blackberries can all make dressings beyond decadent.

Instructions

Here are your instructions. Take a look at your calendar and set a three-day period when you know you'll have time to dedicate to one preparation of a salad per day. You don't have to make your salad at night—you can make it at lunch or even breakfast, or any time of the day you find free time. You can also prepare both the core ingredients and the dressing ahead of time and combine them when you're ready to eat.

The recipes I've included here have been strategically developed, so make sure you make all of them—it's only three days of your life! And make sure you do them in order. The first salad is a foundational recipe, using plenty of common ingredients, like radishes and mint. Along with it is a fundamental dressing that you'll make enough of to use with Day Two's salad. Day Two's salad is a little more interesting, using a deliciously bitter, lesser-known green called frisée along with basil and apple. This is flavor combining at its best. The third is a personal favorite and a guaranteed crowd-pleaser. This Orange & Arugula Salad not only showcases an oil-free dressing, but it introduces the flavor of umami (by using Eastern condiments like miso and soy sauce) into our Reset experience, a flavor that adds a whole new level of depth to salads. It's definitely a recipe that makes you take a bigger leap, in exchange for big rewards.

By the way, all of these salads are easily portable and can be eaten on the go. Pack the salad in one container and the dressing in another container, so you can drizzle it on top just before you eat.

TIPS & TOOLS for EACH DAY

Day One

Welcome to your first day of overhauling salad! Rest assured that after these three days, you will have a brand new love for this staple dish.

Today you will try the first salad—the Peach, Romaine, and Radish Salad. You'll be able to find almost all of these ingredients at your local grocery with the exception of fresh peaches—if they aren't in season, your store may not carry them. If this is the case, you can substitute pears, raspberries, strawberries, or even mango or papaya for the peach. If you can't find romaine, try a prewashed mixed green salad package or any other lettuce. Remember, salads are all about being impromptu and using what's available.

If you usually eat salad for lunch, making it in the morning and bringing it along with you to work may be a good option. As you're making it, think about how the ingredients work together from a texture and flavor perspective. The romaine is slightly sweet, the celery adds crunch, the radishes add further crunch and some bitterness, while the mint adds freshness and a unique coolness.

Make sure that the romaine and mint aren't too wet after you rinse and dry them. If you don't have a salad spinner, it's best to blot out all the extra water using paper towels.

Take care in making the dressing, as it's a classic recipe you can use not only over the course of this Reset, but for the rest of your life if you like it. If you don't have a whisk or a glass bottle with a tight lid, use anything that you may have lying around your kitchen that you can shake a liquid in.

It's always best to taste salad dressing as you go—not only to see if it needs adjustment, but also to get a sense of how dressings should taste and give you something to compare with store-bought varieties. Keep in mind that my salad dressings are on the less oily side, so my recipes tend to taste more vinegary. If you like your dressings less vinegary, just add more olive oil, but do it in small increments. Note how this salad dressing combines the flavors of spicy (black pepper), sweet (balsamic), and sour (vinegar/lemon).

Remember, you can opt to make the dressing days in advance if you want to save time. It stores well in the refrigerator. Just give it a good shake before you use it! And don't dress your salad until the moment you're about to eat the first forkful. If you dress too early, you'll be left with limp greens and an unappealing-looking salad—too wet and too flat.

As you enjoy your salad, check in with yourself and your taste buds. What flavors are you tasting? How does it compare with the salads you've been used to eating? What does the mint do to your senses? How does the peach contrast with the radish? Savor each bite and this new sensory experience.

Day Two

Today you will make the second recipe, the Basil, Lettuce, and Apple Salad. Like yesterday's recipe, this one combines a fruit with an herb and greens.

You should be able to find all these ingredients at the supermarket, with the possible exception of frisée, which is a variety of endive, and a member of the daisy family, with curly, pale green leaves. Frisée, which means "curly" in French, is a beloved ingredient in French cuisine. It is slightly bitter and often used in mesclun mixes. If you can't find it, you may use arugula, escarole, endive, or another salad green of your choice. Just make sure that the green you end up using is a bitter, not a sweet-tasting, one.

There are two main reasons why I enjoy bitter greens like frisée in my salads. The first is flavor. When you contrast the bitterness of greens with the sweetness of fruits and vegetables, your forkful ends up being more dynamic and delicious, as each ingredient helps balance the other. Generally speaking, we're compromising our taste experience by not adding more bitterness to our regular foods. Salads like this one give us a chance to do so. Also, bitter greens—radicchio, dandelion leaves, kale, collards, arugula—tend to be

Dressings That Are Dominated by Oil

Something that has always bothered me about typical salad dressings is the ratio of oil to vinegar, which is usually four-to-one. With this ratio, salad dressings become too oily, which not only weighs down what's underneath but also drowns out flavor. Too much oil takes away from the crisp flavors of lemon juice, vinegar, and mustard. And worse, if refined, processed oils are used—as opposed to cold-pressed oils—even more flavor goes missing. When preparing my recipes below, you'll notice that I rely more on vinegars and less on oils and veer closer to a one-to-one ratio at times, depending on the other ingredients involved.

much more nutrient-dense than sweet greens and other vegetables. In traditional Chinese medicine, they are thought to aid in digestion.

As you start to taste this recipe, home in on the bitterness you experience from the frisée—it is very inviting.

Note in this recipe the use of basil, considered the "king of herbs." Basil is my hands-down favorite herb. It has the perfect shape and texture both for visual appeal and to tear, it's gorgeously sweet, and it's beautifully fragrant. It takes salads to a new level. If you're buying it a few days in advance of your recipe making, make sure to store it in your crisper drawer or in a glass filled with water, like flowers in a vase. It will last longer this way.

Today, you might want to start sharing your newfound salad knowledge with friends and ask them how they define salad. Do they see it as a sacrifice? Do they know that the use of herbs and fruits in salad is fair game and makes salads much more delectable?

At the end of this day, reward yourself for getting this far and being so open-minded with ingredients and your palate.

Day Three

I've saved the best salad recipe for last. Today's recipe helps us redefine salad by bringing in an array of cherished ingredients popular in Japanese cuisine: shoyu, miso, and mirin. These are staple condiments in Japan. Shoyu and mirin are known as the yin and yang of basic seasoning. Shoyu is the Japanese version of soy sauce, and is made by brewing soy-beans with wheat in a fermentation process. It has a rich, umami flavor and is the most popular condiment in Japan.

Miso comes in a paste form—usually in a small package in the refrigerated section of your grocery store near the tofu and other Asian food items. Depending on the variety, it can taste sweet, savory, earthy, or salty. Miso is wonderfully high in protein, vitamins, and minerals. Remember when I demonstrated this recipe to my audience at the farmers' market in San Francisco? Most of the praise I received was for the dressing, which gets its creaminess from the miso, the secret ingredient.

> When you're choosing a dressing at a salad bar, instead of reaching for the processed Ranch or Thousand Island, try a simple drizzling of olive oil and balsamic vinegar with a pinch of salt and pepper.

Mirin has a sweet flavor, so when paired with shoyu and miso, it performs an essential balancing function. Mirin is a rice wine similar to sake but sweeter and with a lower alcohol content. It's used to create teriyaki sauce and is one of the reasons behind the sweet flavor we get when eating sushi rice.

Although this recipe calls for only tablespoons of these condiments, don't worry about the investment you make in buying full bottles. You'll have no problem using up the bottle in the future. Mirin and shoyu (along with some finely minced ginger) make a delectable seasoning for steamed veggies and marinades for fish, for example. And the miso paste can be used to make a simple miso soup.

I originally developed this recipe with kumquats, not oranges. As kumquats are usually hard to find, I added the option of oranges. But keep in mind that if you do end up finding kumquats, try using them instead—they take this salad over the top!

As you enjoy this final salad recipe, take the time to reflect on all the new flavors you've experienced over the last seventy-two hours—the sweetness and freshness of herbs, the umami, the sweetness of peaches and apples, and how they all work so well in combination.

If you have some time today, take a stroll down the salad-dressing aisle and scan the ingredients on the labels. How many ingredients can you pronounce? Think about how the "tomatoes" and "garlic" on these ingredient lists are in no way fresh. How many ingredients do you even recognize as derived from real foods rather than from processing?

At the end of this third day, congratulate yourself on being adventurous. Realize how easy it is to make your own dressing and reward yourself for becoming empowered.

After the Reset

Bravo! This Reset experience has likely left an indelible impression on you. After reading about the origins and modern inadequacies of salad, then getting the opportunity to make tantalizing salads and dressings with your own two hands, you now realize that the way our society defines salad is wrong. This Reset has given you the chance to take time out to properly reassess salad, redefine it, and reimagine it.

You have a whole new skill set now. You know how to prepare salads that take advantage of the wondrous flavors of WAMP foods and in a way that utilizes ingredient combining to maximize flavor. Most important, you know that the tastiest salad dressings can be made in minutes in the comfort of your own kitchen; there's no need to relinquish this power to Kraft or Newman's Own. You've successfully resurrected a lost art form: salad-making. And you now know that dressing is meant for just that: dressing, not drowning.

Now, when you're at a restaurant or cafeteria buffet bar and a dressing label says "Thousand Island," you have a much better idea of what's in it. The mystery associated with salads and dressings has been banished. You're now behind Oz's curtain!

As you move ahead and return to the normal rhythms of your daily life, keep some of the following tips in mind to help keep you on your path:

- When you're choosing a dressing at a salad bar, instead of reaching for the processed Ranch or Thousand Island, try a simple drizzling of olive oil and balsamic vinegar with a pinch of salt and pepper, and a squeeze of lemon.

- Keep my 80/20 Rule in mind. Aim for adhering to the principles of this Reset 80 percent of the time, and for the remainder, give yourself some leeway. If you're stuck at an important work dinner and your salad has arrived at the table drowned in a heavy processed dressing, so be it. If you don't have the time to shop or chop and you

Surprising Salad Suggestions

Here are some ingredients and combinations you may not have considered but should! These make excellent additions to salad mélanges.

- Roasted red peppers
- Large pieces of roasted squash (kabocha squash is my all-time favorite!)
- Yesterday's leftover dinner protein (chicken, salmon, beef, beans, etc.)
- Cooked brown rice or quinoa
- Combining herbs (basil + mint, basil + cilantro)
- Lemon or orange zest
- Purslane
- Shaved fennel
- Any hard cheese (I like to use sheep's cheese)
- Pan-fried tempeh or tofu
- Cooked lentils (I prefer green or Puy lentils)

must go to the neighborhood salad bar, that's OK too. Do what you have to do, but be aware, ask questions, and avoid bad choices when you can.

- When you're at home and want to make a salad but feel you don't have enough of the right ingredients, think again. Take a second look in your crisper drawer, and be brave enough to put together creative combinations of whatever fruits and vegetables you have on hand. Believe me, you'll be surprised with the end result. Remember, salad making is like playing tennis with a huge racket—it's very forgiving with a high success rate.

- Don't forget to continue to experiment. After this Reset is over, continue using different herbs, like parsley and cilantro, in your salads. Cilantro is a personal favorite of mine. It adds exceptional flavor and freshness. Consider unusual fruits and greens, whole grains and proteins too! My typical lunch salad usually consists of chicken, grass-fed beef, or tempeh, along with some rice, baby greens, and whatever veggies I can find in my fridge, along with a homemade dressing. It's beyond divine!

YOUR SALAD RESET GROCERY LIST

- ☐ 1 head romaine lettuce
- ☐ 1 bunch mint
- ☐ 1 peach (or any stone fruit in season or fruit of your choice, e.g., raspberries, strawberries, pears)
- ☐ 1 bunch celery
- ☐ 1 bunch radishes
- ☐ Fresh-ground pepper
- ☐ Organic honey (raw if possible)
- ☐ Balsamic vinegar
- ☐ White wine vinegar
- ☐ Dijon mustard
- ☐ Extra-virgin olive oil
- ☐ 2 Fuji or Granny Smith apples
- ☐ 1 lemon
- ☐ 1 small head butter lettuce

- ☐ 1 bunch basil
- ☐ 1 small head frisée or radicchio or bitter green of your choice
- ☐ 1/4 c pecans
- ☐ Manchego cheese, or hard/firm sheep's cheese (optional)
- ☐ 1 small head Chioggia radicchio
- ☐ 1 package prewashed baby arugula
- ☐ 1/4 c walnuts
- ☐ 4 oranges or c of kumquats plus 1 orange
- ☐ 1 package shiro miso or white miso
- ☐ 1 bottle mirin
- ☐ 1 bottle brown rice vinegar
- ☐ 1 bottle shoyu

Peach, Romaine & Radish Salad
with Balsamic Vinaigrette

I love this dish because it brings together so many unique ingredients and flavors that we don't usually associate with salads: mint, celery, bitter radishes, and sweet honey. Having a recipe for a brilliant balsamic vinaigrette in the back of your pocket is

SERVES: 4
TOTAL TIME: 15 MINUTES

INGREDIENTS
- 1 large head romaine, end of stalk removed, sliced into bite-sized pieces
- Mint leaves from 5–6 stems of mint, torn
- 1 peach, sliced lengthwise into thin wedges (or any stone fruit in season or fruit of your choice, e.g., raspberries, strawberries, pears)
- 3 stalks celery, white portion removed, sliced once down the middle lengthwise, then thinly sliced widthwise into 1/4 inch-thick pieces
- 4–5 small radishes, halved and very thinly sliced
- 5 full turns fresh ground pepper, or 1/8 teaspoon ground pepper (optional)

INGREDIENTS FOR BALSAMIC VINAIGRETTE
- 2–3 tsp organic honey
- 4 tsp balsamic vinegar
- 2 tsp white wine vinegar
- 2 tsp Dijon mustard
- 2 tbsp plus 2 tsp extra-virgin olive oil

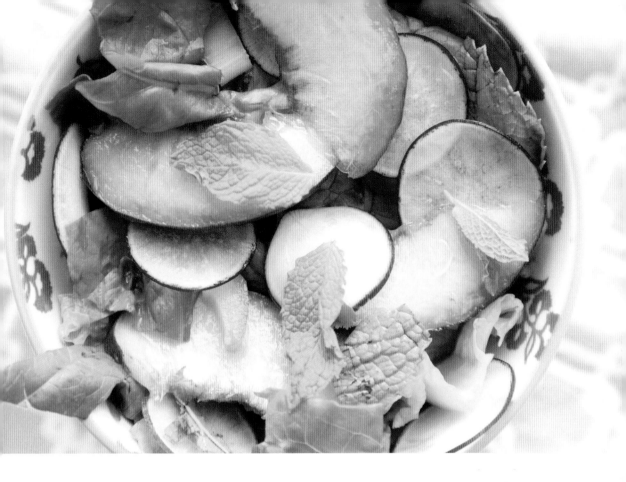

life-altering, seriously. This kind of dressing has so much flavor and depth and works well with a variety of salads. Best of all, you don't need to go to the grocery store but once in order to whip up this dressing for months on end—all the ingredients can last for eons in your fridge and pantry.

PROCEDURE

1. Add all the salad ingredients to a large salad bowl and toss.

2. In a small mixing bowl, whisk together all the dressing ingredients. Pour half of the dressing over the salad and toss to fully coat. If you'd like more dressing, add the rest.

Note: As this dressing is also used in Day Two's recipe, you may opt to double it and save half of it for use tomorrow.

Basil, Lettuce & Apple Salad
with Balsamic Vinaigrette

WAMP salad can't get better or faster than this. Incorporating fruits into salads along with powerfully aromatic herbs like basil—my favorite—changes the game. By incorporating black pepper, walnuts, apples, basil, and cheese, you're guaranteed

SERVES: 4
TOTAL TIME: 15 MINUTES

INGREDIENTS

- 1 1/2 organic Fuji apples or Granny Smith apples (or apple of your choice), cored, thinly sliced from root to stem
- Few squeezes fresh lemon juice
- 5 c butter lettuce leaves, rinsed, patted dry, torn (one small head)
- 1 small head frisée or radicchio, or bitter green of your choice
- 2–3 sprigs basil, rinsed, patted dry, leaves torn
- 1/4 c pecans coarsely chopped
- 5 turns fresh-ground pepper or 1/8 tsp ground pepper
- Manchego cheese or hard sheep's cheese, shaved to taste (optional)

INGREDIENTS FOR BALSAMIC VINAIGRETTE

- 2–3 tsp organic honey
- 4 tsp balsamic vinegar
- 2 tsp white wine vinegar
- 2 tsp Dijon mustard
- 2 tbsp plus 2 tsp extra-virgin olive oil

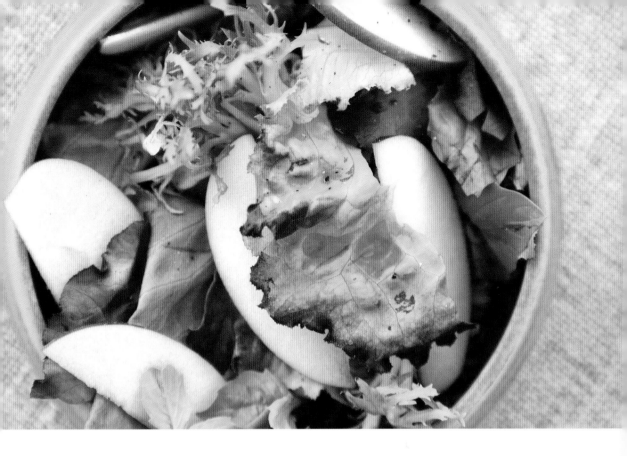

to find naturally sweet, savory, crunchy (from the walnuts), and spicy flavors with each bite—a foodie's dream come true.

PROCEDURE

1. Place the apples into large salad bowl and add the lemon juice. Stir to coat. (Lemon juice prevents apples from oxidizing and turning brown.)

2. Add remaining ingredients and toss.

3. In a small mixing bowl, using a whisk, prepare the dressing by combining all the ingredients, whisking in the olive oil last to properly emulsify.

4. Pour the dressing over the salad and toss to thoroughly coat. Transfer the salad to a salad plate and enjoy immediately.

Note: Using cheese is optional. If you choose to use it, it adds a lot of flavor and contrasts well with the sweetness of the apple and basil. Use a vegetable peeler to shave a small block.

Orange (or Kumquat) & Arugula Salad

with Miso Dressing

This salad will awaken your taste buds and senses with a powerful combination of complex flavors and fragrances—all from nourishing WAMP ingredients. It also proves that some of the best dressings need not contain a drop of oil.

SERVES: 4
TOTAL TIME: 20 MINUTES

INGREDIENTS

- 1/4 head Chioggia radicchio (looks like a small purple cabbage), core removed, thinly sliced
- 4 c prewashed baby arugula
- 25 basil leaves (about 6 sprigs), washed and patted dry, gently torn
- Fresh-ground pepper, about 1/8 to 1/4 teaspoon or about ten turns of peppermill
- 1/4 cup walnuts, coarsely chopped
- Firm sheep's cheese, shaved, to taste
- 1–1 1/2 c organic oranges, cut into segments (supreme) (about 3 oranges) or 3/4 c kumquats, very thinly sliced

INGREDIENTS FOR DRESSING

- Juice of 1 organic orange
- 3 tbsp shiro miso or white miso
- 1 tbsp mirin
- 1 tbsp brown rice vinegar
- 1 tsp shoyu

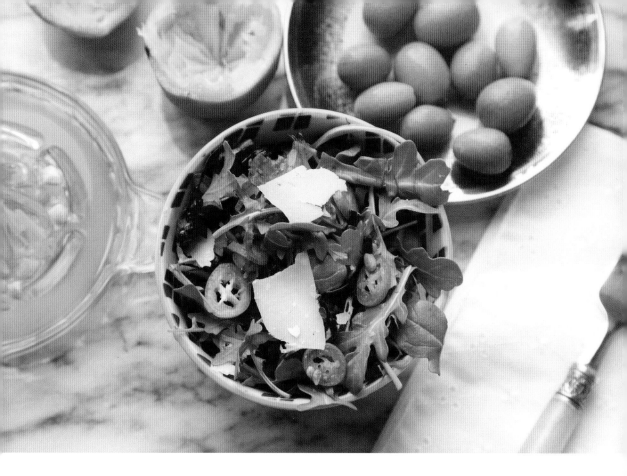

PROCEDURE

1. Combine the greens, ground pepper, and walnuts in a large salad bowl and gently toss.

2. Combine all the dressing ingredients in blender or Vitamix and blend until fully incorporated. Pour dressing in 1/4 cup increments over the salad (taste as you go), and gently toss to coat the greens evenly. There may be dressing left over.

3. Divide among four bowls, and garnish with several orange segments and shaved cheese. Enjoy.

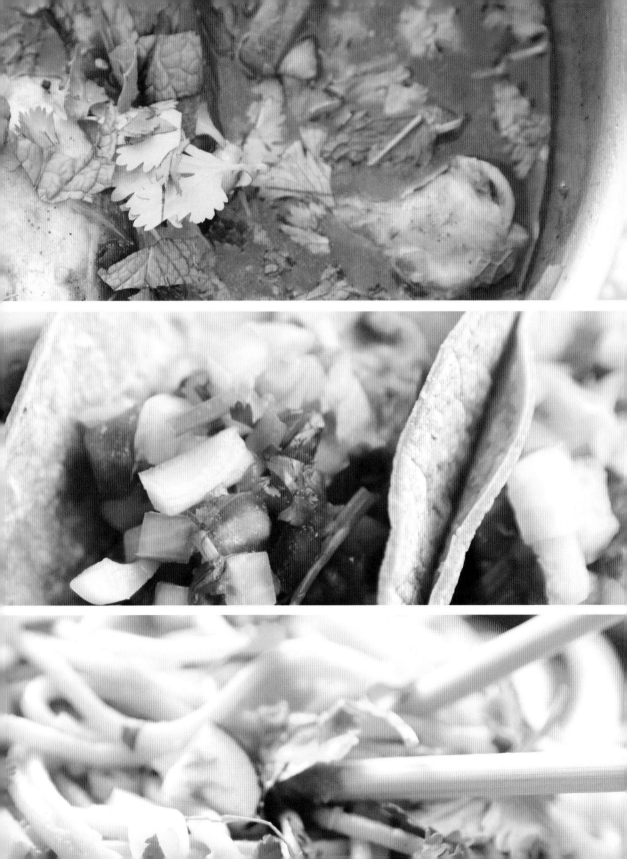

Take-Out
RESET

An unopened bottle of ketchup. A jar of pasta sauce, about a quarter full. A carton of Tropicana Pure Premium. Skim milk. That was all I had in my refrigerator during most of my twenties. Between a demanding Wall Street job, socializing, catching some zzz's, and everything else, my life was busy—too busy to cook.

My savior was take-out. It was a no-brainer. I'd pick up the phone, give somebody my credit-card number, and in less than an hour I'd have pad thai, tandoori chicken, or pasta e fagioli at my front door, all neatly packaged in boxes, complete with utensils and plenty of napkins. Dinner couldn't have been easier.

I thought that ordering dinners from someone else was the greatest thing since sliced bread. I didn't waste time cooking—or cleaning. I ate food, all kinds of glorious global cuisines, prepared authentically by "experts"—much better than anything I could muster myself.

"To go," which accounts for more than half the food we buy from restaurants—dinner being the most popular take-out meal—is akin to what we believe is eating perfection: fast, fun, delectable, and efficient. What more could we want?

271

> Think of eating take-out food as akin to eating a cupcake. It's strategically packaged to look attractive and dazzle the senses.

A lot more. Take-out, which just so happens to be a novel habit in the history of human eating patterns, has done a serious number on us. We think it couldn't be more delicious, yet it can. We believe it's somewhat healthy when it's not.

Take-out is in the business of making a profit—and that's not a simple task. It costs on average a little over $700,000 to open a restaurant, and studies by an Ohio State University associate professor indicate that about 60 percent of restaurants close in their first three-to-five years of operation. To keep costs low and keep us coming back for more, restaurants are motivated to cut corners by using lower-quality ingredients that prey on our biological weakness for salt, fat, sugar, and refined flour. Like the processed foods we buy at the grocery store, much of take-out is designed to make us crave it and to desensitize our taste buds. Even worse, unlike processed foods at the supermarket that come with ingredient lists and labels, take-out food doesn't give anything away.

On top of all this, it's not as authentic as we'd like to believe. Ask any Italian, Chinese, or Greek friend what he thinks of the average Americanized take-out versions of his native dishes and you'll likely get a shake of the head. Many of those dolmades, samosas, and pasta primaveras don't paint a true picture of reality.

The truth is, we don't need to rely on take-out. We can, quite easily, cook great versions of our favorite take-out meals right at home, food that is healthier and much tastier than what comes out of a back kitchen at a Chinese restaurant. In fact, according to a 2013 report released by the USDA's Economic Research Service, food prepared away from home, including take-out and delivery, tends to be lower in nutritional quality than food we cook ourselves and reduces overall diet quality among adults and children.

I'm not suggesting we need to quit dining out or ordering in. That's far from realistic, and wouldn't be enjoyable at all. I mean, who wants to stay at home cooking all the time?

What I'm suggesting instead is that we reset our relationship with take-out so we get to know it better. Let's understand its drawbacks and learn what our WAMP alternatives are. That's what this special Reset is all about: redefining and reimagining take-out. Let's begin!

Take-Out Nation: What We Need to Know About Take-Out Food

When did we start relying on the delivery and pick up of our meals anyway? This grand transformation took root only a little over a half century ago, in the 1950s, the first decade of rock-and-roll.

Before this, we didn't rely so heavily on others for supper. Turning over the reins of dinner preparation for convenience began in earnest with the launch of the TV dinner in 1953. With this frozen ready-made meal, Americans enjoyed a "home-cooked" dinner while watching *I Love Lucy* in the comfort of their living-room armchairs and little to no work in the kitchen. As women joined the workforce and home appliances like toasters and microwave ovens made their way into homes, the trend of eating conveniently evolved from the TV dinner to restaurant dining, to microwave meals, to at-home delivery. In just one generation of Americans, we've managed to eat in an entirely different way from the last, and the thousands of generations previous. Today we manage to obtain more than 30 percent of our calories from food prepared away from home (which includes take-out fare), accounting for 41 percent of our food dollar. Households that represent the highest 20 percent of incomes spend nearly half their food budget on foods made by others.

If there's one thing we're misunderstanding in our nascent "ordering in" culture, it's this: Restaurants are competitive businesses—they're part of a $660.5 billion industry. Most of them aren't putting out hot, boxed, tasty meals solely to nourish and support the long-term health of their customers—that just wouldn't make economic sense in the current marketplace. Although many chefs and restaurateurs get into the business because of their love of good food and the creativity that comes with preparing and serving it, they're also business people who need to sell their food to help pay their rent, taxes, wait staff, and other overhead costs to stay afloat.

There are many tricks of the trade in the restaurant business when it comes to ingredients. Some operations, not just fast-food but full-service restaurants as well, end

> ## Then and Now
>
> In 1955, the same year the Brooklyn Dodgers beat the New York Yankees in the World Series, only about a quarter of the money we spent on food went to eating at restaurants. Today, we spend nearly double that! What's more, well over half the food we buy at these restaurants we eat in our homes, in our cars, or in our offices. In 2006, the typical American ate 81 meals in restaurants but ordered 127 meals as take-out.

up cutting corners by using lower-quality and processed ingredients instead of WAMP ingredients because it's better for their bottom line and easier. As we've learned, processed ingredients are usually cheaper than fresh, are easier to procure, stay shelf-stable longer, and exploit our cravings with refined and exaggerated amounts of refined salt, sugars, and fats (from both animal and plant sources).

That's why most take-out food comes with generous amounts of saltiness, sweetness, and oily richness. If you think about it, no Chinese delivery is short on sodium-rich soy sauce; no steak sandwich is presented without a salty-sweet marinade on the side. Few pasta dishes come without an oily marinara; salads are almost guaranteed to come with overly oily dressings; the average take-out pizza is accompanied by small pools of oil wading inside crispy upturned slices of hot pepperoni, not to mention the traces of oil that come standard at the bottom of the cardboard delivery box it came in.

As a trained chef and recipe developer, I'm intimately involved with flavor: how to manipulate it, enhance it, and maximize it. And when I taste the average take-out, although it may be pretty delicious, I know I'm not getting top-quality, WAMP flavor. Instead, I'm getting flavor in cheap, fake ways. Remember what we discussed in the Salt Reset chapter? We talked about how salt is used to make bland foods or stale ingredients taste better, especially when fresh ingredients are more expensive or difficult to obtain. For example, take-out fare may use extra salt to boost flavor in a sauce instead of herbs like fresh thyme, oregano, or basil. Sometimes it's that extra salt that makes your spring roll taste incredible or your sweet-and-sour pork taste delish, and you may not even

> ## Healthy Fast Food: Not Always an Oxymoron
>
> This Reset doesn't seek to demonize all restaurant take-out food. There are plenty of establishments all over America—more popping up every year—that serve nourishing, delicious food based on WAMP ingredients. I've partnered with the Eat Well Guide to give you a curated guide to some of the best take-out fare you can find. Go to eatwellguide.org to find options near you.

realize it. Surprisingly, based on a 2012 report from the USDA, full-service restaurants use more salt in their meals than even fast food.

Food scientists know the power of fat in flavoring too; they know that fat can enhance flavor by changing a food's mouthfeel, taste, and aroma (it can change its creaminess, appearance, and overall palatability too). But we don't have to be scientists to understand that. We know butter makes a baked potato taste ten times better and olive oil does much the same thing for a piece of bread. So there's a good reason why we often find miniature oil spills at the bottom of most pasta sauces or curry dishes. In many instances, fat—especially processed fat like vegetable oil—makes low-quality food taste better. That's why everything take-out is drowned in it, from French onion soup to pasta pomodoro.

As you can see, restaurants aren't just offering foods that help support their bottom line, they are also developing menus based on what we as customers *demand*. According to U.S. government research, take-out customers rank "taste" as the most important food attribute—higher than "nutrition" and "convenience."

Don't Ask, Don't Tell?

We have no idea what's happening in those kitchens that turn out our take-out. Unlike the food we buy from the grocery store, most of our restaurant meals come with no labels, no information, no trail. We don't know how much salt went into our dish, how the ingredients were prepared, or the amount of added sugar.

Is the chicken Super WAMP? Where did they get the salad greens? Are they using sea salt or refined salt? WAMP oil or processed oils? Are they making steak sauce from scratch or using a bottled brand that's been sitting on the shelf for years? Did they bake the bread fresh or have it shipped in?

We don't ask; they don't tell us. Menus don't explain much. There's no mention of provenance or process. We relinquish the choice of ingredients and preparation of our dinner to strangers in a kitchen we'll never see.

The Grass Ain't Greener

Let's say you're a sucker for a chicken korma dish from your neighborhood Indian take-out place. You crave it like clockwork, maybe once a week. The exotic spices, the savory masala sauce, the perfectly succulent chicken chunks, the heavenly aromas. Now you know the truth: Your take-out korma dish isn't made in the way you imagine. The cooks are overly generous with processed oils, which they use to make the masala sauce and to fry the spices. Salt is added not once, but a few times. The naan or roti that's served with the korma comes from refined white flour. Unless otherwise stated, the yogurt is most likely from factory-farmed animals, as is the chicken.

The chefs may use few fresh vegetables, which means they're using more salt and oil to make up for lost flavor. I know what you're thinking: "My friendly neighborhood restaurant isn't doing things the way I would, but it tastes so good!"

I dare you to take a crack at the korma in your own home. Instead of using a processed oil, choose a higher-quality olive or coconut oil. Instead of refined roti or naan, buy a whole-grain version from the grocery store, if available. In other words, choose WAMP ingredients. Get chicken that's fresh and from sustainable sources. The same goes with yogurt. Throw in more fresh vegetables like carrots and peas as well as the fresh cilantro you picked up on the way home from work. Skip the fried onions. Follow a simple recipe and in the end, you'll see! Your korma will taste crazy good, so much better than the take-out version.

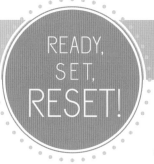

Now that you've learned the pitfalls of take-out, it's time to experience healthier, tastier, WAMP alternatives right at home. Are you ready to embark on the final 3-Day Reset? Like all those that came before it, this Reset helps us fall in love with healthy food. Over the next three days, you'll have the chance to make, taste, and explore your own versions of take-out based on WAMP ingredients.

Just as with the Breakfast and Salad Resets, we will change how we enjoy this fixture in our lives. Please keep your mind and senses open and welcome to change. Many of us believe that cooking international dishes is mysteriously hard and nearly impossible—so difficult that we tend to cop out and order take-out instead. We become anxious about using rarefied ingredients like miso, turmeric, and cardamom. That's normal. But this Reset will empower us to be brave and forge ahead. That's the revolutionary part of it. Remember, it's just three days and you can do *anything* in three days!

Instructions

For this Reset, you'll want to set aside three consecutive evenings to prepare and eat the following dinner recipes, one recipe each night. Because we are a take-out nation that prefers to indulge in international flavors, I've picked recipes that represent three of the most popular ethnic cuisines—Indian, Mexican, and Chinese—to give you the chance to realize just how simple it is to make these types of dishes.

You can find most of the ingredients in these recipes in the international foods section of your grocery store. For the chicken in the second recipe, I recommend finding pasture-raised or USDA organic chicken. Although the spices and Eastern seasonings might seem expensive or a poor investment, know that spices last for six months to a year and that having these ingredients on hand will motivate you to explore more international recipes after this Reset is over.

During this seventy-two-hour period, you'll abstain from all restaurant dinner dining (in-house or to-go). Granted, this might not be easy. Many of us have business dinners, family dinners, holiday dinners, and other commitments that prevent us from cooking and eating at home in the evenings. But for this Reset, do your best to find a period in your calendar that allows you the free time. Remember, you're doing this only once. Give it your all! If it means cooking some of the recipes in advance, that's fine.

You'll also want to take note that these recipes won't taste the same to everyone. Depending on how much you rely on take-out and processed foods, your taste buds might be more desensitized than others.

TIPS & TOOLS for EACH DAY

Day One

Today's recipe is one I believe should be in everyone's culinary arsenal. Wait until you see how easy and delicious it is to make a healthy, delicious version of the fast-food taco!

As you're pulling this recipe together, you'll see how simple it is to source everything—from the beans to the oregano to the salsa ingredients. How does the cilantro smell? What about the aroma that emanates from your saucepan as you're cooking the black beans? Take the time to let your senses be aroused. That's what cooking with our own two hands is all about. If you can't find the mango at your grocery store, try using peaches or canned or fresh pineapple. Both make great substitutes.

As you're shopping for your tacos, the most important ingredient to find is the corn tortillas. This is the type of tortilla that is authentic to Mexican cuisine, not the wheat tortillas we are used to eating these days. Corn tortillas have a wonderfully unique flavor and aroma, with a crunchier, thicker texture than wheat tortillas.

When you sit down to eat, savor the salsa and guacamole. Note how fresh the flavors are in comparison to bottled salsas—or even the salsa and guacamole you eat at restaurants. WAMP ingredients, made fresh by you, always offer better flavor.

If you have leftovers from tonight's meal, you can easily store them. The beans will last for several days. The guacamole and salsa will last a day or two at most.

As you enjoy this fantastic home-cooked meal, think about how rewarding it is to know what's going into your mouth. You chose the ingredients. You prepared the food. You know where the flavor is coming from.

Day Two

Today you'll be making a simple chicken curry.

As you enjoy your meal, notice how this Indian dish compares with those you've eaten at Indian restaurants in the past. You'll likely realize that this homemade version has a lot less oil. You'll notice that it tastes fresher too. Check in with your body afterward. Do you feel lighter than usual?

If your dish tastes slightly underseasoned, add more sea salt *in pinches*. Taste. Remember that if your taste buds are very used to take-out and restaurant fare, they're probably slightly desensitized. If that's the case, do your best to add potency to the dish in other ways. Try using Tabasco sauce to add to its spiciness, or more cilantro to pick up flavor.

Day Three

This last recipe transports us to the Eastern world. Remember: Our palates are meant to experience all five tastes: bitter, sweet, salty, sour, and umami. Because the Western diet is so unbalanced—heavily reliant on sweet and salty—we miss out on experiencing the other three fundamental flavors, specifically umami, which comes from things like soy sauce.

The Chinese Peanut Noodles is not only a cinch to make, but brings together some exquisite flavors by using condiments like rice vinegar and toasted sesame oil, both of which are widely used throughout Asia. You'll realize that they may have been the "mystery ingredients" you had always thought made cooking Chinese, Japanese, or Thai food at home seem so insurmountable.

Your Taste Buds and Your Taste for Take-Out

Many people find that if they change their take-out habits over time (just a few weeks or so), they start to enjoy restaurant fare less and less. That's because when you stop bombarding your taste buds with excessive amounts of salt, oil, sugar, and other processed ingredients, your taste buds wake up!

You'll start craving more nuanced, complex flavor from fresh, high-quality, WAMP meals. Restaurants that serve healthier fare may become your domain. You'll see that the pad thai take-out you used to eat for lunch now seems way too greasy, the portabello mushroom burger way too salty, and the clam chowder swimming in too much cream. You'll become smarter about the food you're eating because your taste buds will regain their natural cravings for WAMP foods.

After the Reset

You have cracked the code on take-out. And you realize that to-go food isn't as delectable as you may have thought. As you graduate from this Reset, feel free to cook these recipes again. Try modifying them. For example, use different fruits in your salsas; add more garlic to your black beans, more spices to your curry, and perhaps some different vegetables to your noodles. Remember, cooking is an art. Practice. Get creative.

You now have an array of skills to help guide you as you continue on the path fully restoring your cravings for healthy foods. As you continue to cook your meals, think of it as if you're catching a fish and cooking it. Realize that it's also the journey, joy, and satisfaction of cooking that makes your food taste so good.

Keep the 80/20 Rule in mind as you move on. If you can cook your dinner or get it from a healthier restaurant in your city 80 percent of the time, there's no need to restrain yourself from eating whatever you want, wherever you want, the remaining 20 percent of the time. Resetting isn't about perfection, it's about making practical, fundamental changes that work in concert with your lifestyle and biology.

YOUR TAKE-OUT RESET GROCERY LIST

- [ ] Coconut oil or extra-virgin olive oil
- [ ] Whole cumin
- [ ] Cinnamon sticks
- [ ] 2 bulbs garlic
- [ ] Cardamom
- [ ] 2 medium to large onions
- [ ] Celery
- [ ] Double-concentrated tomato paste
- [ ] 1 lb ripe organic or heirloom tomatoes or 16 oz can/jar pureed or crushed tomatoes
- [ ] Sea salt
- [ ] Turmeric
- [ ] Chili powder
- [ ] Green bird's eye chili or jalapeño chili
- [ ] 3 limes

- [ ] 2 lbs chicken thighs and/or drumsticks, organic or pasture-raised
- [ ] Ground black pepper
- [ ] 1 bunch cilantro
- [ ] 1 bunch mint
- [ ] 1 15 oz can black beans
- [ ] Apple cider vinegar
- [ ] Dried oregano
- [ ] Ground cumin (if you have a spice grinder at home, grind whole cumin instead)
- [ ] 2 ripe avocados
- [ ] 2 ripe organic or heirloom tomatoes
- [ ] 1 ripe mango
- [ ] Pickled nacho jalapeño peppers
- [ ] 1 package corn tortillas

Black Bean Tacos
with Mango Salsa Fresca

Tacos are a classic Mexican dish, traditionally made with 100 percent corn, not wheat, tortillas wrapped around a filling of various WAMP ingredients including beans, vegetables, minced meat, salsa and guacamole. Tacos are light fare, which is why two or three usually make up one serving size. The recipe below is very simple and is perfect for dinner any day of the week. Most of the ingredients keep well, too, so you can go grocery shopping days in advance.

SERVES: 2 (ABOUT 4–5 TACOS)
TOTAL TIME: 25 MINUTES

INGREDIENTS FOR BLACK BEANS:

- 2 tsp olive oil
- 2 garlic cloves, mashed and chopped
- 1 15-oz can black beans, rinsed and drained
- 1 tbsp apple cider vinegar
- 1/4 tsp dried oregano
- 1/4 tsp ground cumin
- 1/4 tsp sea salt
- 3/4 c cold, filtered water

INGREDIENTS FOR SIMPLE GUACAMOLE:

- 2 ripe avacados
- 4–5 tsp lime juice
- A few generous pinches sea salt
- 2 garlic cloves, mashed and mined

INGREDIENTS FOR SALSA FRESCA:

- 1 medium yellow onion, small dice (about 5 oz)
- 2 small to medium ripe-vine or Roma tomatoes, small dice (about 6 oz)
- 1 ripe mango, small dice (optional)
- 2 tbsp cilantro, chopped
- 2 tbsp pickled nacho jalapeño peppers (or more to taste)

ADDITIONAL:

- 1 package corn tortillas
- Limes, quartered, for garnish

PROCEDURE

1. Heat the oil in a saucepan over low heat. Add the garlic and let it cook for a minute until the fragrant. Add the beans and the remaining ingredients; stir to combine. Bring the water to a boil, then lower the heat to a simmer and cook ten minutes, stirring occasionally.

2. While the beans are cooking, make the guacamole and salsa. For the guacamole, add the avocados to a small mixing bowl along with the garlic, lime juice, and salt and mash it all together. Set it aside. For the salsa, add all the ingredients to another mixing bowl and stir to combine. Set it aside as well.

3. When the beans are done, remove them from the heat. Warm the tortillas using a frying pan—flipping them to make sure both sides become warmed. This should

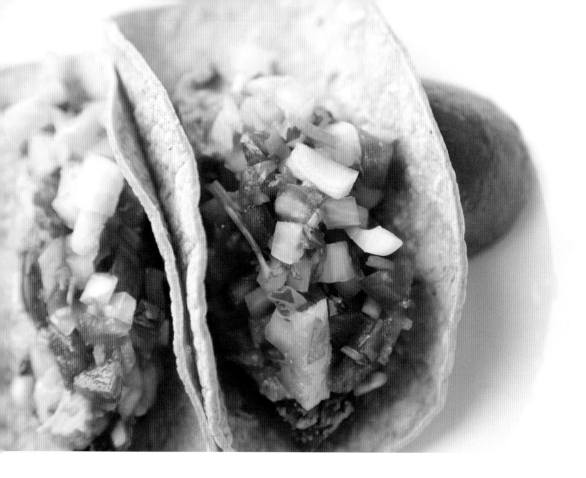

take a few minutes for each tortilla. Then begin to plate your meal. Each taco should receive about a tablespoon and a half of beans, one tablespoon of guacamole, then a heaping tablespoon of salsa on top. Add a few squeezes of lime juice and more chopped jalapeño peppers to taste.

Notes:

• You may double or triple this recipe if you are a family of four, or if you'd like to have enough for leftovers for another day or two.

• I like to use pickled peppers because they're pre-seasoned, easier to handle, and can be stored in your refrigerator. Their heat is also less potent than fresh jalapeño pepper so it's easier to judge how much you want to use!

• If mangoes are not in season or you cannot find them, omit.

Tomato and Onion Chicken Curry

This simple and easy to make chicken curry requires only six spices, some herbs, and bone-in chicken. You may opt to buy the whole leg and ask the butcher to remove the skin for you, then separate the drumstick from the thigh with one easy slice at home. You'll notice I use very little oil, which allows the flavors from the remaining WAMP ingredients to shine through. By combining whole spices like cumin and cloves, ripe tomatoes, and a sprinkling of fresh cilantro and mint, this dish can't help but surprise and enliven your senses.

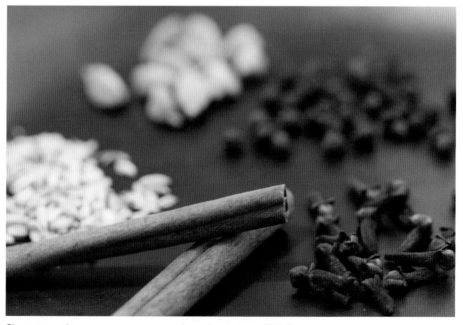

Cinnamon, cloves, peppercorns, and cardamom are WAMP

SERVES: 2–4
TOTAL TIME: 25 MINUTES

INGREDIENTS

- 1 tbsp coconut oil or extra virgin olive oil
- 1 tsp whole cumin seed
- 1 cinnamon stick
- 3 cloves
- 5 cardamom pods, crushed enough for pod to open
- 1 medium to large red onion, thinly sliced or diced
- 1 celery stick, diced
- 1 tbsp double concentrated tomato paste
- 1 lb ripe organic or heirloom tomatoes, pureed (about 4 medium tomatoes)
- 1/2 tsp sea salt
- 1/2 tsp turmeric
- 3/4 tsp chili powder
- 1 inch green birds eye chili or jalapeno chili, finely minced (more to taste)
- 1 1/2–2 lbs chicken thighs and/or drumsticks, organic or pasture raised
- 3/4 to 1 c water
- 1 wedge lime
- 10 turns pepper mill (about 1/4 tsp)
- 1 handful cilantro, bottom stems discarded, chopped
- 1 handful mint, chopped

Tomato and Onion Chicken Curry

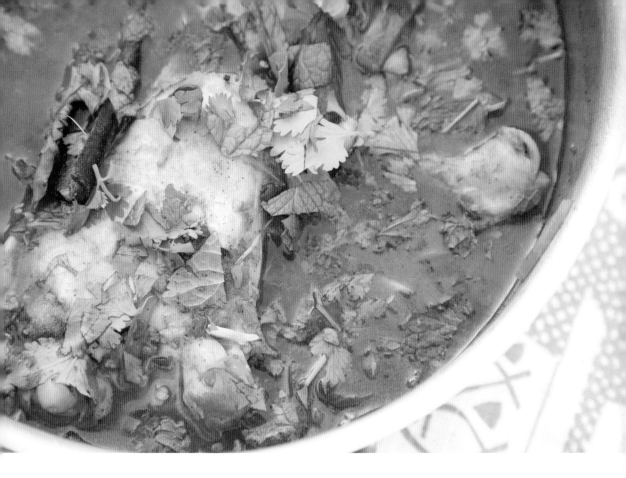

PROCEDURE

1. Heat the oil in a saucepan over medium-low heat. Add the cumin, cinnamon, cloves, and cardamom and cook for a few minutes until the fragrant. Add the onions, celery, and tomato paste and cook a few more minutes until the onions soften.

2. Add the pureed tomatoes and the remaining spices and cook two to three minutes.

3. Add the chicken and enough water to almost cover all the pieces. Bring the liquid to a boil, then lower it to a simmer, cover it, and let it cook for fifteen minutes or until chicken is cooked through.

4. Squeeze the lime juice over the chicken. Taste it and season with pepper and more salt if it is needed. Plate the chicken and garnish it with mint and coriander.

Note: Serve the curry with brown rice and the Raita from the Yogurt Reset chapter.

Chinese Peanut Noodles

This final recipe is quick, WAMP home-cooking at its best. Fresh lime, ginger, garlic, honey, radishes, and cilantro deliver hundreds of wondrous flavor compounds, while Japanese condiments infuse just the right amount of satisfying umami.

SERVES: 4
TOTAL TIME: 15 MINUTES

INGREDIENTS
- 9 oz brown rice noodles or egg noodles (if unavailable, use any linguine-type, whole-wheat noodle)
- 2 tbsp plus 1 tsp toasted sesame oil
- 2 tbsp minced ginger
- 4 tsp minced garlic (about 3–4 cloves)
- 5 tsp shoyu or soy sauce
- 4 1/2 tbsp mirin
- 5 tsp rice wine
- 3 tsp honey
- 3 tbsp lime juice
- 2 1/2 to 3 tbsp organic creamy peanut butter
- Several drops sriracha (hot chili sauce) or Tabasco (or to taste)
- 4–5 scallions, thinly sliced cross wise
- 6 small radishes, quartered, thinly sliced
- Chopped cilantro (for garnish)

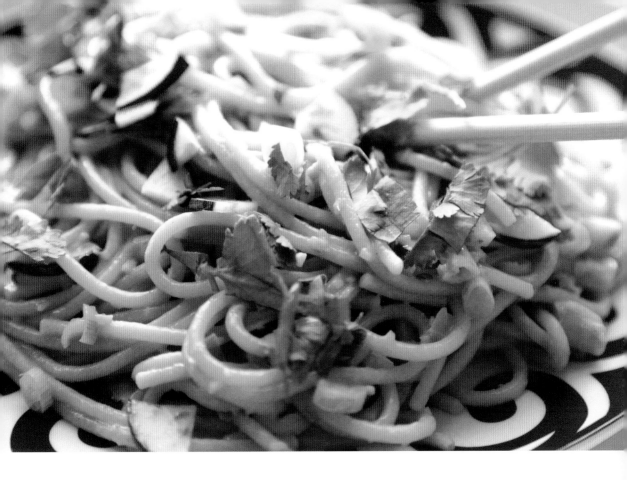

PROCEDURE

1. Bring about 6 cups of water to a boil in a soup pot. Then add the noodles. Cook them for twelve to fifteen minutes. Drain the noodles through a colander and rinse them with cold water. Set them aside in a large serving bowl.

2. In a small saucepan, warm the sesame oil over medium heat. Add the ginger and garlic. Cook them for one minute. Then add all the remaining ingredients including the peanut butter. Stir to incorporate. Cook over low heat until the peanut butter begins to liquefy, a minute or so. Turn off the heat.

3. Add the peanut sauce to the noodles and toss to coat. Add the scallions and radishes and toss again. Plate, garnishing the noodles with fresh cilantro.

Note: If after tasting it, you feel you need more seasoning, try adding small amounts of soy sauce or Sriracha or Tabasco gradually, tasting as you go.

Endotes

What Is a Reset?

The average size of a supermarket / endless aisles are some 40,000 products
"Grocery Stores and Supermarkets." First Research Industry Profile. Last updated December 5, 2005. http://classic.edsuite.com/proposals/proposals_169/88_1_intel_-_grocery_stores.pdf.
See also "Supermarket Industry Overview." Cushman & Wakefield Valuation Service, Retail Industry Group. Last updated in July 2006. http://valuation.cushwake.com/Documents/50905.pdf.

Nearly 70 percent of what we eat comes
See p. xv: Warner, Melanie. *Pandora's Lunchbox: How Processed Food Took Over the American Meal.* New York: Simon & Schuster, 2013.

We're chemically hardwired to be drawn
See chapter 2: Lisle, Douglas, and Alan Goldhamer. *The Pleasure Trap.* ReadHowYouWant.com, 2012.

maximum of three days for us to fully digest
"Digestion: How Long Does It Take?" *Mayo Clinic.* Accessed October 31, 2013. http://www.mayoclinic.com/health/digestive-system/an0089.
See also Martelli, H., Gh Devroede, P. Arhan, C. Duguay, C. Dornic, and C. Faverdin. "Some Parameters of Large Bowel Motility in Normal Man." *Gastroenterology* 75, no. 4 (1978): 612–618.
See also Chan, Yiu-Kay, Ambrose Chi-Pong Kwan, Hon Yue, Yat-Wah Yeung, Kam-Chuen Lai, Justin Wu, Grace Sau-Wai Wong, Chi-Man Leung, Wai-Ching Cheung, and Chi-Kin WongG. "Normal Colon Transit Time in Healthy Chinese Adults in Hong Kong." *Journal of Gastroenterology and Hepatology* 19, no. 11 (2004): 1270–1275.

The Power of WAMP!

Another key attribute of WAMP foods is their deep-rooted connection
Katz, Rebecca, and Mat Edelson. *The Longevity Kitchen.* New York: Random House, 2013.
See also pp. 2–3: Fallon, Sally, and Mary G. Enig. *Nourishing Traditions.* Washington, DC: New Trends Publishing, 1999.

Researchers agree that whole and minimally processed foods
Barr, Sadie B., and Jonathan C. Wright. "Postprandial Energy Expenditure in Whole-Food and Processed-Food Meals: Implications for Daily Energy Expenditure." *Food & Nutrition Research* 54 (2010).
For a good review of the above study, see Kollias, Helen. "Research Review: A Calorie Isn't a Calorie." *Precision Nutrition.* Accessed October 31, 2013. http://www.precisionnutrition.com/digesting-whole-vs-processed-foods
See pp. 37 and 56 in chapters 2 and 3: Fuhrman, Joel. *Eat to Live.* New York: Little, Brown, 2003.
See p. 7: Campbell, T. Colin. *Whole: Rethinking the Science of Nutrition.* Dallas: BenBella Books, 2013.

especially plant-based WAMP foods
See pp. 67, 55, and 74: Fuhrman, Joel. *Eat to Live.* New York: Little, Brown, 2003.

See also Willett, Walter C. "Diet, Nutrition, and Avoidable Cancer." *Environmental Health Perspectives* 103, Supplement 8 (1995): 165.
See also Campbell, Colin T. *The China Study.* Dallas: BenBella Books, 2006.
See also "Teaching the Food System: Food Processing." Center for a Livable Future, John Hopkins Bloomberg School of Public Health. Accessed October 31, 2013. http://www.jhsph.edu/research/centers-and-institutes/teaching-the-food-system/curriculum/_pdf/Food_Processing-Background.pdf.

described as "synergy"
This was addressed by Michael Pollan in a 2007 article in which he used the example of isolating beta carotene by putting it into pill form (what he termed "scientific reductionism"), versus ingesting the entire carrot as a whole food. The conclusion? You didn't get the same benefits from the pill. See Pollan, Michael. "Unhappy Meals." *New York Times Magazine.* Last updated January 28, 2007. http://michaelpollan.com/articles-archive/unhappy-meals/.
This book rethinks the science of nutrition and nutrient extraction from foods, as well as our error in focusing on single nutrients: Campbell, T. Colin. *Whole: Rethinking the Science of Nutrition.* Dallas: BenBella Books, 2013.
See also pp. 55–56: Fuhrman, Joel. *Eat to Live.* New York: Little, Brown, 2003.

According to the FDA, the agency
"Natural and Organic Foods." *Food Marketing Institute Backgrounder*, 2008. http://www.fmi.org/docs/media-backgrounder/natural_organic_foods.pdf?sfvrsn=2.
See also "What Is the Meaning of 'Natural' on the Label of Food?" U.S. Food and Drug Administration. Accessed October 31, 2013. http://www.fda.gov/aboutfda/transparency/basics/ucm214868.htm.
See also McEvoy, Miles. *Use of Natural Flavors.* U.S. Department of Agriculture, Agricultural Marketing Service, National Organic Program, Policy Memorandum 11-1, January 21, 2011.

We know they're uniquely healthy, yet we can't figure out how.
See p. 11: Campbell, T. Colin. *Whole: Rethinking the Science of Nutrition.* Dallas: BenBella Books, 2013.
See also p. 56: Fuhrman, Joel. *Eat to Live.* New York: Little, Brown, and Co., 2003.

scientists have found that humans acquired a sense of taste
See excerpt from *Fast Food Nation* by Eric Schlosser: "Eric Schlosser's Fast Food Nation: Why the Fries Taste Good (Excerpt)." *PBS.* Accessed October 31, 2013. http://www.pbs.org/pov/foodinc/fastfoodnation_03.php.
See also chapter 2: Lisle, Douglas, and Alan Goldhamer. *The Pleasure Trap.* ReadHowYouWant.com, 2012.
See also Yarmolinsky, David A., Charles S. Zuker, and Nicholas J. P. Ryba. "Common Sense About Taste: From Mammals to Insects." *Cell* 139, no. 2 (2009): 234–244.

the potent oils found in an orange peel
"Flavors and Aromas." U.S. Department of Agriculture. Accessed October 31, 2013. http://ars.usda.gov/is/np/alwayssomethingnew/Flavors7.pdf.

Trace minerals, like chromium and manganese
See p. 8: Freye, Enno. *Acquired Mitochondropathy—a New Paradigm in Western Medicine Explaining Chronic Diseases.* Springer, 2012.
See p. 138: Ballantine, Rudolph. *Transition to Vegetarianism: An Evolutionary Step.* Honesdale, PA: Himalayan Institute Press, 1999.

the five basic tastes
NPR segment about the fifth and largely unknown basic taste, umami, on *Morning Edition* that can be found here: Krulwich, Robert. "Sweet, Sour, Salty, Bitter . . . and Umami." NPR: *Morning Edition.* Last updated November 5, 2007. http://www.npr.org/templates/story/story.php?storyId=15819485.
See also Yarmolinsky, David A., Charles S. Zuker, and Nicholas J. P. Ryba. "Common Sense About Taste: From Mammals to Insects." *Cell* 139, no. 2 (2009): 234–244.

"diet-heart hypothesis"
Keys, Ancel, and Josef Brožek. "Body Fat in Adult Man." *Physiological Reviews* 33, no. 3 (1953): 245–325.

had largely backed this work
Initially, the American Heart Association strongly opposed Keys's work, publishing a 15-page report in 1957 denouncing the diet-heart hypothesis. However, in December 1960, the AHA officially adopted the diet-heart hypothesis as their philosophy on heart health, after which *Time* magazine featured Keys on its cover: "Medicine: The Fat of the Land." *Time.* Last updated January 13, 1961. http://content.time.com/time/magazine/article/0,9171,828721,00.html.

you're still not "heart-attack proof"
Mozaffarian, Dariush, Eric B. Rimm, and David M. Herrington. "Dietary Fats, Carbohydrate, and Progression of Coronary Atherosclerosis in Postmenopausal Women." *The American Journal of Clinical Nutrition* 80, no. 5 (2004): 1175–1184. http://www.ncbi.nlm.nih.gov/pubmed/15531663.
See also Mann, George V., and Anne Spoerry. "Studies of a Surfactant and Cholesteremia in the Maasai." *American Journal of Clinical Nutrition* 27, no. 5 (1974): 464–469.
This study, conducted over 8 years on 49,000 women, found virtually identical rates of heart attack, stroke, and other forms of cardiovascular disease in women who followed a low-fat diet and those that did not. See: Howard, Barbara V., JoAnn E. Manson, Marcia L. Stefanick, Shirley A. Beresford, Gail Frank, Bobette Jones, Rebecca J. Rodabough et al. "Low-Fat Dietary Pattern and Weight Change Over 7 Years." *Journal of the American Medical Association* 295, no. 1 (2006): 39–49.
For a review of these and related studies, see Teicholz, Nina. "What If Bad Fat Isn't So Bad?" *Men's Health.* Last updated December 13, 2007. http://www.nbcnews.com/id/22116724/#.UdL9DvnviSp.
See also "Fats and Cholesterol: Out With the Bad, In With the Good." The Nutrition Source, Harvard School of Public Health. Accessed October 31, 2013. http://www.hsph.harvard.edu/nutritionsource/fats-full-story/#Intro.

"disease promoting" and "clearly atherogenic"
Fuhrman, Joel, and Stephen Acocella. "Case Histories: The Atkins Diet." In G. Pugliese, ed., *Disease Proof.* Last updated April 26, 2006. http://www.diseaseproof.com/archives/diet-myths-case-histories-the-atkins-diet.html.

The FDA defines "natural flavoring"
CFR—Code of Federal Regulations Title 21." Food and Drug Administration, U.S. Department of Health and Human Services. Last updated April 1, 2013. http://www.accessdata.fda.gov/scripts/cdrh/cfdocs/cfCFR/CFRSearch.cfm?CFRPart=172&showFR=1&subpartNode=21:3.0.1.1.3.5.

70 percent of our calories
See page xv: Warner, Melanie. *Pandora's Lunchbox: How Processed Food Took Over the American Meal.* New York: Simon & Schuster, 2013.

refined sugar, refined fat (i.e., oils), and refined salt, usually in combination
Moss, Michael. *Salt, Sugar, Fat: How the Food Giants Hooked Us.* New York: Random House, 2013.
See also p. 14: Kessler, David A. *The End of Overeating: Taking Control of the Insatiable American Appetite.* Emmaus, PA: Rodale, 2010.

loading them up with chemicals that tell our brains "this is good, eat me!"
Moss, Michael. *Salt, Sugar, Fat: How the Food Giants Hooked Us.* New York: Random House, 2013.
See chapters 3–7: Kessler, David A. *The End of Overeating: Taking Control of the Insatiable American Appetite.* Emmaus, PA: Rodale, 2010.
See also Lisle, Douglas, and Alan Goldhamer. *The Pleasure Trap.* ReadHowYouWant.com, 2012.

There are nearly 5,000 different kinds in our food supply
International Food Information Council. "Overview of Food Ingredients, Additives & Colors." U.S. Food and Drug Administration, 2010. http://www.fda.gov/downloads/Food/IngredientsPackagingLabeling/ucm094249.pdf.
See p. 171: Warner, Melanie. *Pandora's Lunchbox: How Processed Food Took Over the American Meal.* New York: Simon & Schuster, 2013.

Trained chemists known as "flavorists"
"The Flavorists: Tweaking Tastes and Creating Cravings." *CBS: 60 Minutes.* Last updated September 2, 2012. http://www.cbsnews.com/video/watch/?id=7420280n.
See also Khatchadourian, Raffi. "The Taste Makers: The Secret World of the Flavor Factory." *The New Yorker,* November 23, 2009. http://www.newyorker.com/reporting/2009/11/23/091123fa_fact_khatchadourian.

Food scientists garner degrees from prestigious
Academic Programs: Majors: Food Science." Department of Agriculture, Purdue University. Accessed October 31, 2013. https://ag.purdue.edu/oap/pages/majors.aspx?sid=69.

A 60 Minutes exposé
"The Flavorists: Tweaking Tastes and Creating Cravings." *CBS: 60 Minutes.* Last updated September 2, 2012. http://www.cbsnews.com/video/watch/?id=7420280n.
See also Khatchadourian, Raffi. "The Taste Makers: The Secret World of the Flavor Factory." *The New Yorker,* November 23, 2009. http://www.newyorker.com/reporting/2009/11/23/091123fa_fact_khatchadourian.

Processed foods don't contain the same amount of nutrients
For a good review of nutrient-depleted foods, see Hyman, Mark. "The Last Diet You Will Ever Need." *Huffington Post: Healthy Living.* Last updated June 3, 2012. http://www.huffingtonpost.com/dr-mark-hyman/food-industry_b_1559920.html.

imprinted into our neural circuitry through modifications to our genetic code
Freeman, Kevin B., and Anthony L. Riley. "The Origins of Conditioned Taste Aversion Learning: An Historical Analysis."

Conditioned Taste Aversions: Neural and Behavioral Processes (2008): 9–36.

See also p. 12: Lisle, Douglas, and Alan Goldhamer. *The Pleasure Trap.* ReadHowYouWant.com, 2012.

clinically "addictive," similar to drug addiction

Moss, Michael. "The Extraordinary Science of Addictive Junk Food." *New York Times Magazine.* Last updated February 20, 2013. http://www.nytimes.com/2013/02/24/magazine/the-extraordinary-science-of-junk-food.html?pagewanted=all.

Langreth, Robert, and Duane D. Stanford. "Fatty Foods Addictive as Cocaine in Growing Body of Science." *Bloomberg: Personal Finance.* Last updated November 2, 2011. http://www.bloomberg.com/news/2011-11-02/fatty-foods-addictive-as-cocaine-in-growing-body-of-science.html.

They change the sensitivity of our taste buds

Overberg, Johanna, Thomas Hummel, Heiko Krude, and Susanna Wiegand. "Differences in Taste Sensitivity Between Obese and Non-Obese Children and Adolescents." *Archives of Disease in Childhood* 97, no. 12 (2012): 1048–1052.

For a review of this study, see Sifferlin, Alexandra. "Study: Obese Kids Have Less Sensitive Taste Buds." *Time Health.* Last updated September 20, 2012. http://healthland.time.com/2012/09/20/study-obese-kids-have-less-sensitive-taste-buds/.

Katz, David. "Chicken, Egg, and Taste Buds." *Huffington Post.* Healthy Living. Last updated September 23, 2012. http://www.huffingtonpost.com/david-katz-md/healthy-eating_b_1904033.html.

Dr. David Katz also has a very good book on sensory-specific satiety: Katz, David. *The Flavor Point Diet: The Delicious Breakthrough Plan to Turn Off Your Hunger and Lose the Weight for Good.* Emmaus, PA: Rodale Books, 2005.

Katz, David. "My Conversation with Michael Moss: Bullies, Bodies, and the Body Politic." *Huffington Post.* Healthy Living. Last updated March 1, 2013. http://www.huffingtonpost.com/david-katz-md/food-industry-health_b_2775984.html

Moss, Michael. "The Extraordinary Science of Addictive Junk Food." *New York Times.* Last updated February 20, 2013. http://www.nytimes.com/2013/02/24/magazine/the-extraordinary-science-of-junk-food.html?pagewanted=all.

Moreover, peer-reviewed scientific studies have found

See chapter 2: Contento, Isobel. *Nutrition Education: Linking Research, Theory, and Practice.* Burlington, MA: Jones & Bartlett Learning, 2010.

See also Drewnowski, Adam, Julie A. Mennella, Susan L. Johnson, and France Bellisle. "Sweetness and Food Preference." *Journal of Nutrition* 142, no. 6 (2012): 1142S–1148S. http://www.ncbi.nlm.nih.gov/pubmed/22573785.

that the more our culture becomes acclimated to processed

Lisle, Douglas, and Alan Goldhamer. "How to Escape *The Pleasure Trap*!" Joel Fuhrman. Accessed October 31, 2013. http://www.drfuhrman.com/library/article16.aspx.

Select Additional Sources

Dunn, Rob. "Human Ancestors Were Nearly All Vegetarians." *Scientific American.* Last updated July 23, 2012. http://blogs.scientificamerican.com/guest-blog/2012/07/23/human-ancestors-were-nearly-all-vegetarians/

Matthews, Ruth H., Pamela R. Pehrsson, and Mojgan Farhat-Sabet.

"Sugar Content of Selected Foods: Individual and Total Sugar." *Home Economics Research Report* (1987).

Pollan, Michael. *The Omnivore's Dilemma: A Natural History of Four Meals.* New York: Penguin, 2006.

Sugar Reset

twenty-two teaspoons of sugar

Johnson, Rachel K., et al. "Dietary Sugars Intake and Cardiovascular Health: A Scientific Statement from the American Heart Association." *Circulation* 120, no. 11 (2009): 1011–1020.

13 percent of our total calories

Ervin, R. Bethene, Ph.D., R.D., and Cynthia L. Ogden, Ph.D., M.R.P. "Consumption of Added Sugars Among U.S. Adults, 2005–2010." *NCHS Data Brief* 122 (2013): 1–8.

Humans need sugars, actually

See p. 30: Popkin, Barry. *The World Is Fat: The Fads, Trends, Policies, and Products That Are Fattening the Human Race.* New York: Avery Trade, 2009.

as far back as the Neolithic period

Crane, Eva. *The Archaeology of BeeKeeping.* Ithaca, NY: Cornell University Press, 1983.

sweetener par excellence

See p. 29: Tannahill, Reay. *Food in History.* New York: Crown Publishing Group, 1989.

date or fig syrup, or grape juice

See p. 29: Tannahill, Reay. *Food in History.* New York: Crown Publishing Group, 1989.

Possibly as far back as 1200 BC

See p. 8: Engfer, Lee. *Desserts Around the World.* Minneapolis: Lerner Publishing Group, 2004.

"tables laid with sweet things, syrup, canes to chew"

P. 496: Toussaint-Samat, Maguelonne. *A History of Food.* Oxford: Blackwell Publishing, 2009.

"foray into the valley of the Indus" / "honey without bees."

Pg. 496: Toussaint-Samat, Maguelonne. *A History of Food.* Oxford: Blackwell Publishing, Ltd., 2009.

the Gupta Dynasty (circa AD 500) uncovered a way

See p. 311: Adas, Michael. *Agricultural and Pastoral Societies in Ancient and Classical History.* Philadelphia: Temple University Press, 2001.

The Indians called this sarkara, the Greeks called it "solid honey,"

See p. 497: Toussaint-Samat, Maguelonne. *A History of Food.* Oxford: Blackwell Publishing, 2009.

"worth its weight in silver"

See p. 498: Toussaint-Samat, Maguelonne. *A History of Food.* Oxford: Blackwell Publishing, 2009.

By the 1700s, this separation became de rigueur / "sugarloaf"

See the About Refined Sugar section: "FAQs: Candy." Food Timeline. Accessed October 23, 2013. http://www.foodtimeline.org/foodcandy.html

For a detailed discussion of the process of cutting up sugarloaf with sugar nips, see p. 139: David, Elizabeth. *English Bread and Yeast Cookery*. Middlesex: Penguin, 1977.

By the mid-1800s, a centrifugal machine
One of the first people to apply a mechanical centrifuge in the process of separating sugar from molasses was David Weston, in 1852 at a sugar factory in Hawaii. See p. 138: Galloway, J. H. *The Sugar Cane Industry: An Historical Geography from Its Origins to 1914*. Cambridge: Cambridge University Press, 2005.

Boston Sugar Refinery
Kimball, Christopher. *Fannie's Last Supper: The Meal of the Century*. New York: Random House, 2010.

Sugar refining soon became an industry
"How Sugar is Refined—The Basic Story." *Sugar Knowledge International*. Accessed October 23, 2013. http://www.sucrose.com/lref.html.
See also Augstburger, Franz, et al. "Mango." In *Organic Farming in the Tropics and Subtropics,* 2nd ed. Gräfelfing: Naturland e.V., 2001.
See also "Sugar." In *Cambridge World History of Food*. Edited by Kenneth F. Kiple and Kriemhild Coneè Ornelas. Cambridge: Cambridge University Press, 2000. http://www.cambridge.org/us/books/kiple/sugar.htm.
See also "Refining and Processing Sugar: Consumer Fact Sheet." Sugar Association. Accessed October 23, 2013. http://www.western-sugar.com/pdf/Refining%20and%20Processing%20Sugar.pdf.

In 1745 it was discovered that sugar / imports in 1813
See p. 504: Toussaint-Samat, Maguelonne. *A History of Food*. Oxford: Blackwell Publishing, 2009.

sugar-beet production in the United States today is genetically modified
USDA Economic Research Service. "Adoption of Genetically Engineered Crops in the U.S." Data set. Last updated July 8, 2013. http://www.ers.usda.gov/datafiles/Adoption_of_Genetically_Engineered_Crops_in_the_US/alltables.xls.
NPR broadcast a segment in 2010 about genetically engineered sugar beets on *All Things Considered*: Charles, Dan. *Sugar Beet Beatdown: Engineered Varieties Banned*. Podcast audio. *NPR: All Things Considered*. Accessed October 23, 2013. http://www.npr.org/templates/story/story.php?storyId=129891767.

Its story begins in the 1970s
For the amount of HFCS added to soft drinks from 1970 to 2000, see Bray, George A. "How Bad Is Fructose?" *American Journal of Clinical Nutrition* 86, no. 4 (2007): 895–896.
HFCS is less expensive than sucrose for several reasons, including sugar production quotas, U.S. corn subsidies, and an import tariff on foreign sugar. See also Pollan, Michael. *The Way We Live Now: The (Agri)Cultural Contradictions of Obesity*. New York Times Magazine, October 12, 2003. http://www.nytimes.com/2003/10/12/magazine/12WWLN.html.

alteration of chemical bonds
Visuri, Kalevi, and Alexander M. Klibanov. "Enzymatic Production of High Fructose Corn Syrup (HFCS) Containing 55% Fructose in Aqueous Ethanol." *Biotechnology and Bioengineering* 30, no. 7 (1987): 917–920.
See also Hyman, Mark, M.D. "5 Reasons High Fructose Corn Syrup Will Kill You." Dr. Hyman. Last modified May 4, 2013. http://

drhyman.com/blog/2011/05/13/5-reasons-high-fructose-corn-syrup-will-kill-you/#close.

evenly among sugar cane, sugar beets, and corn derived sweeteners.
See p. 4: Moss, Michael. *Salt, Sugar, Fat: How the Food Giants Hooked Us*. New York: Random House, 2013.

Common Processed Sugars Added to Our Foods
"Sugars 101." Nutrition Center, American Heart Association. Last updated March 11, 2013. http://www.heart.org/HEARTORG/GettingHealthy/NutritionCenter/Sugars-101_UCM_306024_Article.jsp.

other 30 percent from drinks
Ervin, R. Bethene, Ph.D., R.D., and Cynthia L. Ogden, Ph.D., M.R.P. "Consumption of Added Sugars Among U.S. Adults, 2005–2010." *NCHS Data Brief* 122 (2013): 1–8.

In 1822, American adults ate
Schomer, Stephanie. "Sugar Shock: 4 Things You Didn't Know About Your Diet." *O: The Oprah Magazine*, January 2013. http://www.oprah.com/health/Health-Facts-About-Sugar-Sugar-and-Diets/4.

Maple syrup, for example, has a flavor chemistry
"FAQ." Cornell Maple Sugar Research & Extension Program. Accessed October 23, 2013. http://maple.dnr.cornell.edu/FAQ.htm.

Select Additional Sources
O'Connor, Anahad. "Really? Most of the Added Sugar in Our Diets Comes From Sugary Drinks." *New York Times*. Last updated May 6, 2013. http://well.blogs.nytimes.com/2013/05/06/really-most-of-the-added-sugar-in-our-diets-comes-from-sugary-drinks/.
Renton, Alex. "Coca-Cola's Sugar Problem." *Guardian*. Last updated January 18, 2013. http://www.theguardian.com/lifeandstyle/wordofmouth/2013/jan/18/coca-cola-sugar-problem.
Moßhammer, Markus R., Florian C. Stintzing, and Reinhold Carle. "Evaluation of Different Methods for the Production of Juice Concentrates and Fruit Powders From Cactus Pear." *Innovative Food Science and Emerging Technologies* 7, no. 4 (2006): 275–287.
"FAQ." *American Sugar Alliance*. Accessed October 23, 2013. http://www.sugaralliance.org/faq.html.

Salt Reset
"not worth his salt"
"History of Salt." Salt Institute. Accessed October 24, 2013. http://www.saltinstitute.org/salt-101/.

It's often said that much of Napoleon's army . . . the British Empire in 1947.
Regarding salt deficiency in Napoleon's army, see: Zimmermann, Michael B. "Research on Iodine Deficiency and Goiter in the 19th and Early 20th Centuries." *Journal of Nutrition* 138, no. 11 (2008): 2060–2063.
For the role of salt in India's struggled for independence, see pp. 181–182: Bakshi, S. R. *Indian Freedom Fighters: Struggle for Independence*. New Delhi, India: Anmol Publications, 2002.

40 percent over the last four decades
"Sodium, Salt, and You." *Harvard Women's Health Watch*. Last updated June 2009. http://www.health.harvard.edu/newsletters/Harvard_Womens_Health_Watch/2009/November/sodium-salt-and-you.

Agricultural Research Service. "What We Eat in America." U.S. Department of Agriculture. Last updated 2010: www.ars.usda.gov/services/docs.htm?docid=18349.

Our ancestors have been
See chapter 14: Toussaint-Samat, Maguelonne. *A History of Food.* Oxford: Blackwell Publishing, 2009.
See also pp. 179–181: Tannahill, Reay. *Food in History.* New York: Crown Publishing Group, 1989.

Neolithic people settled in places
See p. 417: Toussaint-Samat, Maguelonne. *A History of Food.* Oxford: Blackwell Publishing, 2009.

Roman colonization of Palestine
See p. 420: Toussaint-Samat, Maguelonne. *A History of Food.* Oxford: Blackwell Publishing, 2009.

both heavily reliant on salt, particularly processed (refined) salt
Most Americans get 75% of their daily sodium intake from prepared foods. See "Salt and Sodium." The Nutrition Source, Harvard School of Public Health. Accessed October 24, 2013. http://www.hsph.harvard.edu/nutritionsource/salt-and-sodium/?utm_campaign=socialflow&utm_source=twitter&utm_medium=social.
The 75% statistic comes from Brown, Ian J., Vanessa Candeias Tzoulaki, and Paul Elliott. "Salt Intakes Around the World: Implications for Public Health." *International Journal of Epidemiology* 38, no. 3 (2009): 791–813.
According to the CDC, most of the sodium we ingest comes from packaged, processed, store-bought, and restaurant foods. See "Sodium and Food Sources." *Center for Disease Control & Prevention.* Accessed October 24, 2013. http://www.cdc.gov/salt/food.htm.
The CDC cites the following peer-reviewed study: Mattes, R. D., and D. Donnelly. "Relative Contributions of Dietary Sodium Sources." *Journal of the American College of Nutrition* 10, no. 4 (1991): 383–393.

trace minerals
"Celtic Sea Salt." Health Freedom Resources. Accessed October 26, 2013. http://healthfree.com/celtic_sea_salt.html
See also Kuhnlein, Harriet V. "The Trace Element Content Of Indigenous Salts Compared With Commercially Refined Substitutes." *Ecology of Food and Nutrition* 10, no. 2 (1980): 113–181.
"Sea Salt Vs. Table Salt." American Heart Association. Last updated September 11, 2013. http://www.heart.org/HEARTORG/Conditions/HighBloodPressure/PreventionTreatmentofHighBloodPressure/Sea-Salt-Vs-Table-Salt_UCM_430992_Article.jsp.
For a good discussion on the processing of salt, see "HimalaSalt." HimalaSalt. Accessed October 26, 2013. http://www.himalasalt.com/index.php?page=product&display=7.
See also pp. 48–49: Fallon, Sally. *Nourishing Traditions.* Washington, DC: NewTrends Publishing, Inc., 1999.

calcium silicate
By law, the FDA permits no more than 2%, by weight, of this anti-caking agent in foods. See "CFR–Code of Federal Regulations Title 21." Food and Drug Administration, U.S. Department of Health and Human Services. Last updated April 1, 2013. http://www.accessdata.fda.gov/scripts/cdrh/cfdocs/cfCFR/CFRSearch.cfm?CFRPart=172&showFR=1&subpartNode=21:3.0.1.1.3.5.

70 percent of our calories from processed foods
Warner, Melanie. "Pandora's Lunchbox." Melanie Warner. Accessed October 26, 2013. http://melanierwarner.com/pandoras-lunchbox/.
See also Warner, Melanie. *Pandora's Lunchbox: How Processed Food Took Over the American Meal.* New York: Simon & Schuster, 2013.

half of the money we spend on food
Stewart, Hayden, Noel Blisard, and Dean Jolliffe. *Let's Eat Out: Americans Weigh Taste, Convenience, and Nutrition.* No. 59411. U.S. Department of Agriculture, Economic Research Service, 2006.

Nutrition Facts box in 1984
"Appendix B, Government Initiatives and Past Recommendations of the National Academies, the World Health Organization, and Other Health Professional Organizations." In Jane E. Henry and Christine L. Taylor, eds. *Strategies to Reduce Sodium Intake in the United States.* Washington, DC: National Academies Press, 2010.

More than 3,300 milligrams
"Sodium and Food Sources." Centers for Disease Control & Prevention. Accessed October 24, 2013. http://www.cdc.gov/salt/food.htm.

salt in the ancient world was around 250 milligrams
He, F. J., and G. A. MacGregor. "A Comprehensive Review on Salt and Health and Current Experience of Worldwide Salt Reduction Programmes." *Journal of Human Hypertension* 23, no. 6 (2008): 363–384.

According to the Harvard School of Public Health
"Salt and Sodium." The Nutrition Source, Harvard School of Public Health. Accessed October 24, 2013. http://www.hsph.harvard.edu/nutritionsource/salt-and-sodium/?utm_campaign=socialflow&utm_source=twitter&utm_medium=social.

Manufacturers know that salt enhances flavor
See NPR review of Moss's *Salt, Sugar, Fat*: Boeschenstein, Nell. "How the Food Industry Manipulates Taste Buds with Salt, Sugar, Fat." NPR: The Salt. Last updated February 26, 2013. http://www.npr.org/blogs/thesalt/2013/02/26/172969363/how-the-food-industry-manipulates-taste-buds-with-salt-sugar-fat.

food scientists have found a whole new set of ways that salt
For a good discussion on what salt can do for processed foods, see pp. 281–283 and 288: Moss, Michael. *Salt, Sugar, Fat: How the Food Giants Hooked Us.* New York: Random House, 2013.
See also "Appendix B, Government Initiatives and Past Recommendations of the National Academies, the World Health Organization, and Other Health Professional Organizations." In Jane E. Henry and Christine L. Taylor, eds. *Strategies to Reduce Sodium Intake in the United States.* Washington, DC: National Academies Press, 2010.

balance the metallic aftertastes
See "Sodium and Salt: Health Concerns and Regulatory Status." White Paper. AIB International, Manhattan, KS, 2008. https://www.aibonline.org/researchandtechnical/white%20papers/Sodium-Jan2008.pdf.

Salt is used to make sugary foods more sugary
See p. 288: Moss, Michael. *Salt, Sugar, Fat: How the Food Giants Hooked Us.* New York: Random House, 2013.

salt suppresses bitterness in food
Agrawal, Anurag A., and Richard Karban. "Salt Enhances Flavour by Suppressing Bitterness." *Nature* 387 (1997): 563.

activation of certain sweet receptors
Yee, Karen K., Sunil K. Sukumaran, Ramana Kotha, Timothy A. Gilbertson, and Robert F. Margolskee. "Glucose Transporters and ATP-Gated K+ (KATP) Metabolic Sensors Are Present in Type 1 Taste Receptor 3 (T1r3)–Expressing Taste Cells." *Proceedings of the National Academy of Sciences* 108, no. 13 (2011): 5431–5436.

25 percent of our sodium intake
"Nine in 10 U.S. Adults Get Too Much Sodium Every Day." *Centers for Disease Control and Prevention.* Last updated February 7, 2012. http://www.cdc.gov/media/releases/2012/p0207_sodium_food.html.

National restaurant chains are some of the worst culprits
"Heart Attack Entre?es and Side Orders of Stroke: The Salt in Restaurant Meals Is Sabotaging Your Health." *Center for Science in the Public Interest.* Accessed October 26, 2013. http://cspinet.org/new/pdf/cspirestaurantsaltreport.pdf.

taste buds can gradually adjust
See pp. 283 and 295: Moss, Michael. *Salt, Sugar, Fat: How the Food Giants Hooked Us.* New York: Random House, 2013.

Vilhjalmur Stefansson
Stefansson, Vilhjalmur. *Not by Bread Alone.* New York: Macmillan, 1946.

Select Additional Sources
Farley, Thomas A. "Salt Is a Problem; Salt Shakers Are." *New York Times: Room for Debate.* Last updated September 10, 2103. http://www.nytimes.com/roomfordebate/2013/09/10/should-salt-have-a-place-at-the-table/salt-is-a-problem-but-salt-shakers-arent.
Chapters 12 and 13: Moss, Michael. *Salt, Sugar, Fat: How the Food Giants Hooked Us.* New York: Random House, 2013.
O'Connor, Anahad. "'Really?' The Claim Sea Salt Is Lower in Sodium Than Table Salt." *New York Times: Well.* Last updated August 29, 2011. http://well.blogs.nytimes.com/2011/08/29/really-the-claim-sea-salt-is-lower-in-sodium-than-table-salt/.
For a thorough review of the current literature on salt, see Taubes, Gary. "Salt, We Misjudged You." *New York Times.* Last updated June 2, 2012. http://www.nytimes.com/2012/06/03/opinion/sunday/we-only-think-we-know-the-truth-about-salt.html?pagewanted=all.
Tannahill indicates that by now the human race is "genetically programmed" to need salt. See p. 357: Tannahill, Reay. *Food in History.* New York: Crown Publishing Group, 1989.

Wheat Reset

three billion are sold
About 3 billion pizzas are sold in the United States per year, according to the National Association of Pizzeria Operators (NAPO). See "A Slice of Pizza Stats." General Electric. Last updated August 18, 2010. http://pressroom.geappliances.com/news/Pizza_stats_07.

85 billion tortillas
A year 2000 statistic from the Tortilla Industry Association. See p. 7: Steinback, Jyl. *Cook Once, Eat for a Week.* New York: Penguin, 2002.

seventy-five percent
See "Wheat Info." National Association of Wheat Growers. Accessed October 24, 2013. http://www.wheatworld.org/wheat-info/fast-facts/.

20 percent of all calories
See p. 13: Davis, William. *Wheat Belly: Lose the Wheat, Lose the Weight, and Find Your Path Back to Health.* New York: HarperCollins Publishers, 2011.
See also Murphy, Pat. *Plan C: Community Survival Strategies for Peak Oil and Climate Change.* Vancouver: New Society Publishers, 2013.

USDA's radar for compiling
See Table 217: U.S. Census Bureau. "Per Capita Consumption of Major Food Commodities: 1980 to 2009." *Statistical Abstract of the United States* (2012).
See also Lin, Biing-Hwan, and Steven T. Yen. "The U.S. Grain Consumption Landscape: Who Eats Grain, in What Form, Where, and How Much?" *Economic Research Report* 50 (2007).

Around 10,000 BC
See p. 21: Tannahill, Reay. *Food in History.* New York: Crown Publishing Group, 1989.
See also "Ears of Plenty." *Economist.* Last updated December 20, 2005. http://www.economist.com/node/5323362.
See also p. 115: Toussaint-Samat, Maguelonne. *A History of Food.* Oxford: Blackwell Publishing, 2009.

because of calories from wheat
See "Ears of Plenty." *Economist.* Last updated December 20, 2005. http://www.economist.com/node/5323362

Plato's Republic (380 BC)
See p. 125: Toussaint-Samat, Maguelonne. *A History of Food.* Oxford: Blackwell Publishing, 2009.

According to Socrates
See p. 77: Kostigen, Thomas M. *The Big Handout: How Government Subsidies and Corporate Welfare Corrupt the World We Live In and Wreak Havoc on Our Food Bills.* Emmaus, PA: Rodale, 2011.

using millstones
See p. 23: Tannahill, Reay. *Food in History.* New York: Crown Publishing Group, 1989.

It was likely in this way that we were consuming wheat
Food historians generally cite 4000 BC as the year that leavened bread was discovered, but other sources point to archaeological evidence dating to 2000 BC.
See also p. 267: Huang, H. T. *Fermentations and Food Science,* vol. 6. Cambridge: Cambridge University Press, 2000.
See also "FAQs: Bread." Food Timeline. Accessed October 24, 2013. http://www.foodtimeline.org/foodbreads.html.
It is generally thought that bread making was the precursor to ale making. See also pp. 48 and 51–52: Tannahill, Reay. *Food in History.* New York: Crown Publishing Group, 1989.
See also p. 517: McGee, Harold. *On Food and Cooking: The Science and Lore of the Kitchen.* New York: Scribner, 2004.

Chinese around 1700 BC
See p. 170: Toussaint-Samat, Maguelonne. *A History of Food.* Oxford: Blackwell Publishing, 2009.

rotary querns / water mills
See pp. 33 and 41: Lynch, Alban J., and Chester A. Rowland. *The History of Grinding.* Dearborn: SME, 2005.
See also "Invention of the Water Mill." *The Age.* Last updated

March 6, 1948. http://news.google.com/newspapers?nid=1300&dat=19480306&id=M8ATAAAAIBAJ&sjid=Vb8DAAAAIBAJ&pg=7202,3128859.

horsehair
See p. 36: Lynch, Alban J., and Chester A. Rowland. *The History of Grinding.* Dearborn: SME, 2005.

roller mill around 1870
See p. 107: Pollan, Michael. *In Defense of Food.* London: Penguin Books, 2009.

75 percent of phytochemicals are lost
"Nutrition: Whole Grains." Office of Statewide Health Improvement Initiatives, Minnesota Department of Health. Last updated June 2012. http://www.health.state.mn.us/divs/hpcd/chp/cdrr/nutrition/docsandpdf/wholegrainfactsheet.pdf.

so the U.S. government mandated that flour and breads be enriched
Gorton, Laurie. "70 Years and Counting of Enriched Wheat." Baking Business. Last updated September 14, 2011. http://www.bakingbusiness.com/News/News%20Home/Features/2011/9/70%20years%20and%20counting%20of%20enriched%20wheat.aspx?cck=1.

How Wheat is Converted to Flour (Chart)
"Wheat Milling Process." North American Millers' Association. Accessed October 24, 2013. http://www.namamillers.org/education/wheat-milling-process/.

according to the Whole Grain Council
"Whole Grain Statistics." Whole Grains Council. Accessed October 24, 2013. http://wholegrainscouncil.org/node/58/print.

Sadly, less than 2 percent of the wheat flour
Figure based on 1997 data. See p. 1: USDA Office of Communications. *Agriculture Fact Book 1999.* U.S. Department of Agriculture, 2000.

Nabisco Honey Maid Honey Grahams
For nutrition information, see "Nabisco Honey Maid Honey." Snack Works. Accessed October 24, 2013. http://www.snackworks.com/products/product-detail.aspx?product=4400000463.

home baking accounted for 90 percent of flour consumption
"Wheat's Role in the U.S. Diet." USDA Economic Research Service. Accessed October 24, 2013. http://www.ers.usda.gov/topics/crops/wheat/wheats-role-in-the-us-diet.aspx.

including gun puffing and extrusion
See chapter 4, especially pp. 58–64: Warner, Melanie. *Pandora's Lunchbox: How Processed Food Took Over the American Meal.* New York: Simon & Schuster, 2013.
See also Fallon, Sally. "Dirty Secrets of the Food Processing Industry." Weston A. Price Foundation. Last updated March, 2011. http://www.westonaprice.org/modern-foods/dirty-secrets-of-the-food-processing-industry.
See also Chatel, Robert E., Sandy Mui, and Justin A. French. "Expansion of Extruded Cereals With Good Source of Fiber." WIPO Patent 2010051181. Issued May 7, 2010.
See also Newman, Barry. "No Grapes, No Nuts, No Market Share: A Venerable Cereal Faces Crunchtime." *Wall Street Journal.*

Last updated June 1, 2009. http://online.wsj.com/news/articles/SB124381591156970663.

Select Additional Sources
iGrow Wheat: Best Management Practices for Wheat Production
See pp. 22–26: Tannahill, Reay. *Food in History.* New York: Crown Publishing Group, 1989.
Whole Grain Council, http://wholegrainscouncil.org/.
See pp. 99–102: Warner, Melanie. *Pandora's Lunchbox: How Processed Food Took Over the American Meal.* New York: Simon & Schuster, 2013.
Davis, William. *Wheat Belly: Lose the Wheat, Lose the Weight, and Find Your Path Back to Health.* New York: HarperCollins Publishers, 2011.
"Wheat's Role in the U.S. Diet." *USDA Economic Research Service.* Accessed October 24, 2013. http://www.ers.usda.gov/topics/crops/wheat/wheats-role-in-the-us-diet.aspx
Economic Research Service. *The U.S. Grain Consumption Landscape: Who Eats Grain, in What Form, Where, and How Much?* U.S. Department of Agriculture, 2012.

Chocolate Reset
cacahuaquchtl
See p. 515: Toussaint-Samat, Maguelonne. *A History of Food.* Oxford: Blackwell Publishing, 2009.

supposedly gulped
See p. 242: Tannahill, Reay. *Food in History.* New York: Crown Publishing Group, 1989.

Vases used to serve
"Chocolate Art Collections." Museum of Fine Arts, Boston. Accessed October 26, 2013. http://www.mfa.org/sites/default/files/Chocolate_English_web_0.pdf.

tchocoatl
See p. 516: Toussaint-Samat, Maguelonne. *A History of Food.* Oxford: Blackwell Publishing, 2009.

"delightfully unclad virgins"
See p. 517: Toussaint-Samat, Maguelonne. *A History of Food.* Oxford: Blackwell Publishing, Ltd., 2009.

fifty cups of it per day
"Aztec Hot Chocolate." British Museum. Accessed October 26, 2013. http://www.britishmuseum.org/explore/young_explorers/create/aztec_hot_chocolate.aspx.

Veracruz, Mexico, to Seville, Spain, took place in 1585
See p. 217: Freedman, Paul H. *Food: The History of Taste.* London: Thames & Hudson, 2007.

mid-1600s
See p. 518: Toussaint-Samat, Maguelonne. *A History of Food.* Oxford: Blackwell Publishing, 2009.

palace of Versailles in 1682
See p. 518: Toussaint-Samat, Maguelonne. *A History of Food.* Oxford: Blackwell Publishing, 2009.

It wouldn't be until the nineteenth century
See p. 242: Tannahill, Reay. *Food in History*. New York: Crown Publishing Group, 1989.

opened in France around 1824
See p. 519: Toussaint-Samat, Maguelonne. *A History of Food*. Oxford: Blackwell Publishing, 2009.

Back in America, in 1894
See "Our Story." Hershey's. Accessed October 2, 2013. http://www. hersheys.com/our-story.aspx#/the-company.

although this step may get skipped altogether
Sunita De Tourreil, interview with author, Palo Alto, California, September 21, 2013. De Tourreil is the founder of the Chocolate Garage, a chocolate tasting room in Palo Alto, California. See: http://thechocolategarage.com/about.html.

This concoction is then further ground in roller mills
See "The Factory" on the National Confectioners' Association website The Story of Chocolate. Accessed October 27, 2013. http:// www.thestoryofchocolate.com/where/content.cfm?ItemNumber=3304&navItemNumber=3258.

According to the FDA
For citations pertaining to this paragraph, see "CFR–Code of Federal Regulations Title 21." Food and Drug Administration, U.S. Department of Health and Human Services. Last updated April 1, 2013. http://www.accessdata.fda.gov/scripts/cdrh/cfdocs/cfCFR/CFRSearch.cfm?CFRPart=172&showFR=1&subpartNode=21:3.0.1.1.3.5.

chock-full of nourishment
"Heart-Health Benefits of Chocolate Unveiled." Cleveland Clinic. Accessed October 27, 2013. http://my.clevelandclinic.org/heart/prevention/nutrition/chocolate.aspx.
See also Hannum, Sandra M., and John W. Erdman Jr. "Emerging Health Benefits from Cocoa and Chocolate." *Journal of Medicinal Food* 3, no. 2 (2000): 73–75.

although it depends on how the chocolate was processed
The Cleveland Clinic states that best choices are dark chocolate and cacao powder that hasn't undergone Dutch processing: "Heart-Health Benefits of Chocolate Unveiled." Cleveland Clinic. Accessed October 27, 2013. http://my.clevelandclinic.org/heart/prevention/nutrition/chocolate.aspx.
In this piece from the *New York Times*, the darker the chocolate (WAMP chocolate), the more likely it is that it will be higher in flavonoids: Parker-Pope, Tara. "The Problem with Chocolate." *New York Times: Well*. Last updated December 21, 2011. http://well.blogs.nytimes.com/2007/12/21/the-problem-with-chocolate/?_r=0.

flavonoids
Steinberg, Francene M., Monica M. Bearden, and Carl L. Keen. "Cocoa and Chocolate Flavonoids: Implications for Cardiovascular Health." *Journal of the American Dietetic Association* 103, no. 2 (2003): 215–223.

National Confectioners Association's Chocolate Council
"Cacao Percentages." The Story of Chocolate. Accessed October 26, 2013. http://www.thestoryofchocolate.com/Savor/content.cfm?ItemNumber=3454&navItemNumber=3376.

percentage of cacao in a bar
"The Percentages." The Story of Chocolate, website of the National Confectioners' Association. Accessed October 27, 2013. http://www.thestoryofchocolate.com/Savor/content.cfm?ItemNumber=3454&navItemNumber=3376.

1,500 flavors alone
Kuczynski, Alex. "Spellbound by Chocolate." *New York Times*. Last updated February 9, 2006. http://www.nytimes.com/2006/02/09/fashion/thursdaystyles/09CRITIC.html?pagewanted=all.

taste different from chocolate made from beans harvested in Madagascar
John Ferry, CEO, Madecasse Chocolate, phone interview with author, October 2012.

Chocolate flavor also comes from the fermentation and roasting processes
Barringer, Sheryl. "The Chemistry of Chocolate Flavor." Ohio State University. Accessed October 27, 2013. http://library.osu.edu/assets/Uploads/ScienceCafe/Barringer020310.pdf.

Select Additional Sources
Chapter 18: Toussaint-Samat, Maguelonne. *A History of Food*. Oxford: Blackwell Publishing, Ltd., 2009.
"Appendix III: Draft Revised Standard for Cocoa (Cacao) Mass (Cocoa/Chocolate Liquor) and Cocoa Cake (Advanced at Step 8 of the Procedure)" in: *Report of the Codex Committee on Cocoa Products and Chocolate*. Food and Agriculture Organization of the United Nations. Accessed October 27, 2013.
http://www.fao.org/docrep/meeting/005/x8943e/x8943e0e.htm.
"The Bitter Truth Behind the Chocolate in Your Easter Basket." CNN: Eatocracy. Last updated April 4, 2012. http://eatocracy.cnn.com/2012/04/04/slavery-free-chocolate/.
For expert-level information on chocolate and cacao, see this excellent site, specifically the "Chocolate Flavor Profiles" under Chocolate Atlas: C Spot. Accessed October 27, 2013. http://www.c-spot.com/.

Yogurt Reset

Food of the Gods / wild bacteria cultures in the air
See p. 170. Batmanglij, Najmieh. *A Taste of Persia: An Introduction to Persian Cooking*. London: I. B. Tauris, 2007.
See also pp. 27–29: Tannahill, Reay. *Food in History*. New York: Crown Publishing Group, 1989.

Bulgaria is referred to as the "cradle of yogurt."
See p. 341: Freedman, Paul H. *Food: The History of Taste*. London: Thames & Hudson, 2007.
Iran and India
See p. 373: Ayoto, John. *An A to Z of Food and Drink*. Oxford: Oxford University Press, 2002.

Ilya Mechnikov
"Ilya Mechnikov–Biographical." NobelPrize.org. Accessed October 27, 2013. http://www.nobelprize.org/nobel_prizes/medicine/laureates/1908/mechnikov-bio.html.

Genghis Khan purportedly offered yogurt
See p. 87: Weatherford, Jack. *Genghis Khan and the Making of the Modern World*. New York: Random House, 2005.

King François I of France had a nasty case of diarrhea
See pp. 108–109: Toussaint-Samat, Maguelonne. *A History of Food.* Oxford: Blackwell Publishing, 2009.
See also p. 216: Lahtinen, Sampo, Seppo Salminen, Atte Von Wright, and Arthur C. Ouwehand, eds. *Lactic Acid Bacteria: Microbiological and Functional Aspects.* Boca Raton, FL: CRC Press, 2011.

Isaac Carasso
For a fascinating read on the history of Danone, see "The History of Danone" on the company website. Accessed October 27, 2013. http://www.danone.com/en/press-releases/cp-mai-2009.html.
Another great read on the life of Mr. Carasso can be found in this *New York Times* piece: Grimes, William. "Daniel Carasso, a Pioneer of Yogurt, Dies at 103." *New York Times.* Last updated May 20, 2009. http://www.nytimes.com/2009/05/21/business/21carasso.html.

"a traditional Bulgarian preparation assuring a long and healthy life"
See pp. 341–343: Freedman, Paul H. *Food: The History of Taste.* London: Thames & Hudson, 2007.

1947 introduced something that
Grimes, William. "Daniel Carasso, a Pioneer of Yogurt, Dies at 103." *New York Times.* Last updated May 20, 2009. http://www.nytimes.com/2009/05/21/business/21carasso.html.

began operations in the United States in 1942 under the name Dannon
See "Our Heritage." Dannon Company. Accessed October 27, 2013. http://www.dannon.com/pages/rt_aboutdannon_oheritage.html.

"annual book of dairy statistics"—but not until 1989
"Yogurt Added to U.S. Dairy Statistics." *Milwaukee Sentinel.* Last updated May 11, 1990. http://news.google.com/newspapers?nid=1368&dat=19900511&id=NJZQAAAAIBAJ&sjid=uxIEAAAAIBAJ&pg=4764,3618294.
See also Kendall, Don. "Yogurt Makes USDA Statistics Book for the First Time." *Associated Press.* Last updated May 10, 1990. http://www.apnewsarchive.com/1990/Yogurt-Makes-USDA-Statistics-Book-for-First-Time/id-2a7ee700e820732857259f36b55fbec5.

a shocking 400 percent
"Greek Yogurt Surges." *Food Business News.* Accessed October 27, 2013. http://www.foodbusinessnews.net/Resources/Corporate%20Profiles%20Categories/Dairy/Ice%20cream%20sales%20rebound%20Greek%20yogurt%20surges.aspx?cck=1.

fastest-growing segment
Economic Research Service. "Data Set." U.S. Department of Agriculture. Last updated October 23, 2013. http://www.ers.usda.gov/data-products/dairy-data.aspx#.UmBXaWTk94Q.

Secretary of Agriculture to modify USDA guidelines
See press release from New York Senator Gillibrand's office: Gillibrand, Kirsten. "After Meeting With Chobani, Gillibrand-Hanna Urge USDA To Reclassify Greek Yogurt In Nutrition Guidelines." Kirsten Gillibrand News. Last updated August 30, 2012. http://www.gillibrand.senate.gov/newsroom/press/release/after-meeting-with-chobani-gillibrand-hanna-urge-usda-to-reclassify-greek-yogurt-in-nutrition-guidelines.

Stabilizers improve mouthfeel
Benoit de Korsak, phone interview with the author, March 2013.

slapped Dannon for unsubstantiated claims
Bowdler, Neil. "EU Health Food Claims Law Begins to Bite." BBC News Health. Last updated July 6, 2010. http://www.bbc.co.uk/news/10240263.

Dannon had to pony up $35 million on the back of similar charges
Williams, Timothy. "Dannon Settles With F.T.C. Over Some Health Claims." *New York Times.* Last updated December 15, 2010. http://www.nytimes.com/2010/12/16/business/16yogurt.html.

invented in 1971
McGinn, Daniel. "The Great Froyo Gold Rush." *Boston Globe.* Last updated May 26, 2013. http://www.bostonglobe.com/magazine/2013/05/25/pinkberry-orange-leaf-and-more-charting-frozen-yogurt-gold-rush/vZZ5RMe2MVUV6u7g9Eo8tM/story.html.

Select Additional Sources
Mudeva, Anna. "Want to Live 100 Years? Eat Bulgarian Yoghurt." Reuters. Last updated April 27, 2003. http://www.freerepublic.com/focus/f-news/901494/posts.
Aubrey, Allison. "Confusion at the Yogurt Aisle? Time for Probiotics 101." NPR: The Salt. Last updated July 9, 2012. http://www.npr.org/blogs/thesalt/2012/07/09/156381323/confusion-at-the-yogurt-aisle-time-for-probiotics-101.
Barclay, Eliza. "Eternal Yogurt: The Starter That Lives Forever." NPR: The Salt. Last updated May 1, 2011. http://www.npr.org/blogs/thesalt/2012/04/30/151699885/eternal-yogurt-the-starter-that-lives-forever.

Chicken Reset
83 percent of our chicken in whole form / we buy only about 11 percent
"How Broilers Are Marketed." National Chicken Council. Accessed October 27, 2013. http://www.nationalchickencouncil.org/about-the-industry/statistics/how-broilers-are-marketed/.

60 percent of chicken-part purchases
Clark, Melissa. "A Fallen Star of French Cuisine, Restored to Its Silver Platter." *New York Times.* Last updated January 12, 2010. http://www.nytimes.com/2010/01/13/dining/13appe.html?src=tp&_r=0.

95 percent of chicken
Safran-Foer, Jonathan. "The Truth About Factory Farming." Government Accountability Project. Last updated February 22, 2010. http://www.whistleblower.org/press/gap-in-the-news/361.
See also "New Jersey Battles to Protect Pregnant Pigs." ASPCA. Last updated October 22, 2013. http://www.aspca.org/blog/term/farm-animal-cruelty.
See also "Our Story." Compassion in World Farming. Accessed October 27, 2013.
http://www.ciwf.com/our-story/.
The NCC doesn't refer to "factory farms," but instead uses the phrase "vertically integrated" and "production contracts": "Broiler Chicken Industry Key Facts." National Chicken Council. Accessed October 27, 2013. http://www.nationalchickencouncil.org/about-the-industry/statistics/broiler-chicken-industry-key-facts/.

48 percent of chicken sold to us as processed products
"How Broilers Are Marketed." National Chicken Council. Accessed October 27, 2013. http://www.nationalchickencouncil.org/about-the-industry/statistics/how-broilers-are-marketed/.

According to Eric Schlosser

In reference to this section pertaining to McNuggets, please see pp. 139–142: *Fast Food Nation: The Dark Side of the All-American Meal.* Boston: Houghton-Mifflin Harcourt, 2012.

"mechanically separated chicken" (MSC)

Cortez-Vega, William Renzo, Gustavo Graciano Fonseca, and Carlos Prentice. "Effects of Soybean Protein, Potato Starch and Pig Lard on the Properties of Frankfurters Formulated From Mechanically Separated Chicken Meat Surimi-Like Material." *Food Science and Technology International* (2013).

See also Miles, Robert, Scott Anderson, Lassiter Mason, and Juanita Schwartzkopf. "Poultry Processing Economic Review 2012." Focus Management Group. Accessed October 27, 2013. http://www.focusmg.com/white-papers/poultry-processing-economic-review.

since the 1960s

"Mechanically Separated Chicken." National Chicken Council. Last updated May, 2012. http://www.nationalchickencouncil.org/wp-content/uploads/2012/05/Mechanically-Separated-Chicken-May-2012.pdf.

By 2010, poultry had outrun

Bentley, Jeanine. "U.S. Consumption of Chicken Surpasses That of Beef." U.S. Department of Agriculture, Economic Research Service. Accessed October 27, 2013. http://www.ers.usda.gov/amber-waves/2012-september/us-consumption-of-chicken.aspx#.Umb6ABbPV3Y.

Americans eat more chicken

See statistics from the 2012 U.S. Census : "Table 1377: Meat Consumption by Type and Country: 2009–2010." U.S. Census Bureau, *Statistical Abstract of the United States: 2012.* Accessed October 27, 2013. http://www.census.gov/compendia/statab/2012/tables/12s1375.pdf.

83 pounds per person each year

"Per Capita Consumption of Poultry and Livestock, 1965 to Estimated 2014, in Pounds." National Chicken Council. Accessed October 27, 2013. http://www.nationalchickencouncil.org/about-the-industry/statistics/per-capita-consumption-of-poultry-and-livestock-1965-to-estimated-2012-in-pounds/.

football field

See p. 171: Pollan, Michael. *The Omnivore's Dilemma: A Natural History of Four Meals.* New York: Penguin, 2006.

349 pounds by our second birthday

See p. 62: Weber, Karl. *Food, Inc: How Industrial Food Is Making Us Sicker, Fatter, and Poorer–And What You Can Do About It.* New York: Perseus Books Group, 2009.

See also Bittman, Mark. "A Chicken Without Guilt." *New York Times.* Last updated March 11, 2012. http://www.nytimes.com/2012/03/11/opinion/sunday/finally-fake-chicken-worth-eating.html?_r=0.

See also "The Big 6." *Powered by Produce.* Accessed October 27, 2013. http://www.powered-by-produce.com/2009/08/21/the-dirty-six/.

conjugated linoleic acid (CLAs)

See p. 32: Planck, Nina. *Real Food: What to Eat and Why.* New York: Bloomsbury, 2007.

sunlight or a varied diet / have devised fake chicken flavoring

See pp. 171–176: Warner, Melanie. *Pandora's Lunchbox: How Processed Food Took Over the American Meal.* New York: Simon & Schuster, 2013.

57 percent of these at fast-food restaurants

"Retail Grocery Continues to Dominate Chicken Marketing." National Chicken Council. Accessed October 27, 2013. http://www.nationalchickencouncil.org/retail-grocery-continues-to-dominate-chicken-marketing/.

dark meat contains more iron, zinc

"White Meat Vs. Dark Meat." *Chicken Farmers of Canada.* Accessed October 27, 2013. http://www.chicken.ca/health/view/2/white-meat-vs.-dark-meat.

From a health perspective, stocks have

"Broth Is Beautiful." Weston A. Price Foundation website. Accessed October 27, 2013. http://www.westonaprice.org/food-features/broth-is-beautiful.

See also p. 49: Fallon, Sally. *Nourishing Traditions.* Washington, DC: NewTrends Publishing, 1999.

Dubbed "Jewish penicillin"

See p. 32: Planck, Nina. *Real Food: What to Eat and Why.* New York: Bloomsbury, 2007.

Select Additional Sources

"Big Chicken: Pollution and Industrial Poultry Production in America." Pew Environment Group. Accessed October 28, 2013. http://www.pewenvironment.org/uploadedFiles/PEG/Publications/Report/PEG_BigChicken_July2011.pdf.

"Kings of the Carnivores." *Economist.* Last updated April 30, 2012. http://www.economist.com/blogs/graphicdetail/2012/04/daily-chart-17.

Jennings, Holly. "Why Pasture Eggs Taste Better Than Those From Factory Farms." *Boston Globe.* Last updated April 4, 2012. http://www.bostonglobe.com/lifestyle/food-dining/2012/04/03/these-hens-roam-range-and-eat-well/OSNwjSNPj4NsR6hMFr5CCL/story.html.

For an understanding of why pasture chicken taste better, see McKenna, Maryn. "Beyond Factory Farming: An Appetite for Pastured Poultry." *WIRED.* Last updated June 11, 2012. http://www.wired.com/wiredscience/2012/06/pastured-poultry-week/.

See pp. 169–173: Pollan, Michael. *The Omnivore's Dilemma: A Natural History of Four Meals.* New York: Penguin, 2006.

For an understanding of nutrient differences between conventional and pasture chicken, see the following, especially pp. 252–254: Salatin, Joel. *Folks, This Ain't Normal: A Farmer's Advice for Happier Hens, Healthier People, and a Better World.* New York: Center Street, 2012.

Eckblad, Marshall. "Dark Meat Getting a Leg Up on Boring Boneless Breast." *Wall Street Journal.* Last updated April 15, 2012. http://online.wsj.com/news/articles/SB10001424052702304587704577333923937879132.

For information on poultry labeling, see this report: "Meat and Poultry Labeling Terms." Food Safety Information. Food Safety and Inspection Service, U.S. Department of Agriculture. Accessed October 28, 2013. http://www.fsis.usda.gov/wps/wcm/connect/e2853601-3edb-45d3-90dc-1bef17b7f277/Meat_and_Poultry_Labeling_Terms.pdf?MOD=AJPERES.

Beverage Reset

nearly half of the added sugar in our diet comes from drinks
Smith, Travis, Biing-Hwan Lin, and Jong-Ying Lee. "Taxing Caloric Sweetened Beverages: Potential Effects on Beverage Consumption, Calorie Intake, and Obesity." U.S. Department of Agriculture Economic Research Service, Economic Research Report 100 (2010).

Until roughly 9000 BC
Wolf, A., G. A. Bray, and B. M. Popkin. "A Short History of Beverages and How Our Body Treats Them." *Obesity Reviews* 9, no. 2 (2008): 151–164.

2700 BC
See p. 177: Standage, Tom. *A History of the World in 6 Glasses.* New York: Walker, 2006.

using carbonation to create bubbles in 1772
Hooper, J. "History and Ccope of the Fruit Juices and Drinks Industry." *International Journal of Dairy Technology* 37, no. 3 (1984): 101–106.

Coca-Cola's original formulation
"The Recipe." *This American Life.* Accessed October 28, 2013. http://www.thisamericanlife.org/radio-archives/episode/427/original-recipe/recipe.

lime and lemon juice on ocean journeys was mandatory
Cook, G. C. "Scurvy in the British Mercantile Marine in the 19th Century, and the Contribution of the Seamen's Hospital Society." *Postgraduate Medical Journal* 80, no. 942 (2004): 224–229.

juice en masse until the twentieth century
See p. 103: Hooper, J. "History and Scope of the Fruit Juices and Drinks Industry." *International Journal of Dairy Technology* 37, no. 3 (1984): 101–106.

invented until the 1930s
See p. 91: Ohlgren, Schott, and Joann Tomasulo. *The 28-Day Cleansing Program: The Proven Recipe System for Skin and Digestive Repair.* Buffalo, NY: 28 Day Cleansing Program, 2006.

Florida citrus crisis in the 1950s
See p. 57: Popkin, Barry. *The World Is Fat: The Fads, Trends, Policies, and Products That Are Fattening the Human Race.* New York: Avery Trade, 2009.

particularly the orange juice you find in
Hamilton, Alissa. "Freshly Squeezed: The Truth About Orange Juice in Boxes." *Civil Eats.* Last updated May 6, 2009. http://civileats.com/2009/05/06/freshly-squeezed-the-truth-about-orange-juice-in-boxes/.
See also "Why '100% Orange Juice' Is Still Artificial." *Huffington Post:* Food. Last updated September 28, 2011. http://www.huffingtonpost.com/2011/07/29/100-percent-orange-juice-artificial_n_913395.html.

contain just 5 percent juice
"Fuze Beverage." *Walgreens.* Accessed October 28, 2013. http://www.walgreens.com/store/c/fuze-beverage/ID=prod6068181http://www.walgreens.com/store/c/fuze-beverage/ID=prod6068181-product–descriptionNamedTab-product#descriptionNamedTab.

Nearly 85 percent of the tea
"Tea Fact Sheet." *Tea Association of the U.S.A.* Accessed October 28, 2013. http://www.teausa.com/14655/tea-fact-sheet.

In 2010, the average American drank nearly
Zmuda, Natalie. "Bottom's Up." *Adage.* Last updated June 27, 2011. http://adage.com/article/news/consumers-drink-soft-drinks-water-beer/228422/.

sugary drinks exploit our innate weakness for sweetness
McKiernan, Fiona, Jenny A. Houchins, and Richard D. Mattes. "Relationships Between Human Thirst, Hunger, Drinking, and Feeding." *Physiology and Behavior* 94, no. 5 (2008): 700–708.
See also Rolls, Barbara J., Sion Kim, and Ingrid C. Fedoroff. "Effects of Drinks Sweetened With Sucrose or Aspartame on Hunger, Thirst and Food Intake in Men." *Physiology and Behavior* 48, no. 1 (1990): 19–26.
See also Langreth, Robert, and Duane D. Stanford. "Fatty Foods Addictive as Cocaine in Growing Body of Science." *Bloomberg News.* Last updated November 2, 2011. http://www.bloomberg.com/news/2011-11-02/fatty-foods-addictive-as-cocaine-in-growing-body-of-science.html.

"encourage drinking that is not necessarily linked to fluid needs"
McKiernan, Fiona, James H. Hollis, George P. McCabe, and Richard D. Mattes. "Thirst-Drinking, Hunger-Eating; Tight Coupling?" *Journal of the American Dietetic Association* 109, no. 3 (2009): 486–490.
http://www.ncbi.nlm.nih.gov/pubmed/?term=McKiernan F%5Bauth%5D.

Select Additional Sources
Chapter 2: Popkin, Barry. *The World Is Fat: The Fads, Trends, Policies, and Products That Are Fattening the Human Race.* New York: Avery Trade, 2009.
Chapter 20: Toussaint-Samat, Maguelonne. *A History of Food.* Oxford: Blackwell Publishing, 2009.
"Breaking Down the Chain: A Guide to the Soft Drink Industry." *National Policy and Legal Analysis Network to Prevent Childhood Obesity.* Accessed October 28, 2013. http://www.foodpolitics.com/wp-content/uploads/SoftDrinkIndustryMarketing_11.pdf.
"Beverage Industry Terms." *American Beverage Industry.* Accessed October 28, 2013.
http://www.ameribev.org/resources/beverage-industry-terms/.
"Frappuccino." Starbucks. Accessed October 28, 2013. http://frappuccino.com/en-us/products.

Breakfast Reset
About 60 percent of the foods
Langer, Gary. "POLL: What Americans Eat For Breakfast." ABC News. Last updated May 17, 2005. http://abcnews.go.com/GMA/PollVault/story?id=762685.

leading pancake syrup brand
"Original." Aunt Jemima. Accessed October 28, 2013. http://www.auntjemima.com/aj_products/syrups/orginal.cfm.

vanilla-frosted scone from a major coffeehouse
"Petite Vanilla Bean Scone." Starbucks. Accessed October 28, 2013. http://www.starbucks.com/menu/food/bakery/petite-vanilla-bean-scone.

breakfast cereals in a box didn't exist
Warner, Melanie. *Pandora's Lunchbox: How Processed Food Took Over the American Meal.* New York: Simon & Schuster, 2013.

buckwheat ("buckwheats") and cornmeal pancakes ("Indian cakes")
See pp. 229–230: Mariani, John F., ed. *Encyclopedia of American Food and Drink.* New York: Lebhar-Friedman, 1999.

buckwheat—an ancient plant, related to rhubarb
See "Buckwheat–December Grain of the Month." Whole Grains Council. Accessed October 28, 2013. http://wholegrainscouncil.org/whole-grains-101/buckwheat-december-grain-of-the-month.

The first commercially sold, prepared, and packaged
"Aunt Jemima's Historical Timeline." Aunt Jemima. Accessed October 31, 2013. http://www.auntjemima.com/aj_history/.

late 1890s, it was made of a variety of flours
A picture of the box from the 1930s with ingredients can be found here: "A Familiar Face." Scriblets. Last updated March 19, 2012. http://wwwscriblets-bleets.blogspot.com/2012/03/familiar-face.html.

Early settlers used maple syrup
"Indians and the Early Maple Sugaring Process." *New England Maple Museum.* Accessed October 31, 2013. http://www.maplemuseum.com/indians-and-early-maple-sugaring-process.

The original muffins and scones
"Muffins." Food Timeline. Accessed October 31, 2013. http://www.foodtimeline.org/foodfaq2.html#muffins.

Traditional brioche, croissants
"Breakfast Pastries." *Jean-Mark Chatellier's Bakery.* Accessed October 31, 2013. http://www.jeanmarcchatellier.com/breakfast.html.
See also "Brioche." Food Timeline. Accessed October 31, 2013. http://www.foodtimeline.org/foodbreads.html#brioche.

queen of France Marie Antoinette
"The Croissant." France.fr: The Official Website of France. Accessed October 31, 2013. http://www.france.fr/en/gastronomy/croissant.

John Harvey Kellogg experimented with wheat
See p. 56–59: Warner, Melanie. *Pandora's Lunchbox: How Processed Food Took Over the American Meal.* New York: Simon & Schuster, 2013.

the most adulterated breakfast
See chapter 4, "Extruded and Gun Puffed": Warner, Melanie. *Pandora's Lunchbox: How Processed Food Took Over the American Meal.* New York: Simon & Schuster, 2013.

combo meals
Middleton, Ekin. "Starbucks Offers Coffee-Breakfast Combos, Cites Economy." CNN: U.S. Last updated February 9, 2009. http://www.cnn.com/2009/US/02/09/starbucks.offers/.

Salad Reset
somewhere between 4000 and 3000 BC
See p. 185: Toussaint-Samat, Maguelonne. *A History of Food.* Oxford: Blackwell Publishing, Ltd., 2009.
See also Tannahill, Reay. *Food in History.* New York: Crown Publishing Group, 1989.

"best of all salad plants" / Venus slept on a bed of lettuce
See p. 628: Toussaint-Samat, Maguelonne. *A History of Food.* Oxford: Blackwell Publishing, 2009.

Hence salad got its name from the character
See p. 682: Davidson, Alan. *Oxford Companion to Food, 2nd ed.* Oxford: Oxford University, 2006.

salade in French
See p. 628: Toussaint-Samat, Maguelonne. *A History of Food.* Oxford: Blackwell Publishing, 2009.

The Potager du Roi
"Le Potager du Roi." Le Potager du Roi Versailles. Accessed October 31, 2013. http://www.potager-du-roi.fr/site/potager/index.htm.
See also pp. 547–557: See p. 628: Toussaint-Samat, Maguelonne. *A History of Food.* Oxford: Blackwell Publishing, 2009.

The French king apparently had a weakness
See p. 626: Toussaint-Samat, Maguelonne. *A History of Food.* Oxford: Blackwell Publishing, 2009.

In 1924, an immigrant restaurateur
"Caesar Salad." Princeton wiki. Accessed October 31, 2013. http://www.princeton.edu/~achaney/tmve/wiki100k/docs/Caesar_salad.html.

The same decade
"Cobb Salad." Food Timeline. Accessed October 31, 2013. http://www.foodtimeline.org/foodsalads.html#cobb.

in the 1960s when "salad bars,"
Holley, Joe. "Entrepreneur Norman Brinker, 78, Pioneered Casual Dining, Invented Salad Bar." *Washington Post.* Last updated June 10, 2009. http://www.washingtonpost.com/wp-dyn/content/article/2009/06/09/AR2009060903038.html.

Invented in 1952, the original recipe for ranch dressing
Koerner, Brendan. "Ranch Dressing: Why Do Americans Love It So Much?" *Slate.* Last updated August 5, 2005. http://www.slate.com/articles/arts/number_1/2005/08/ranch_dressing.html.
See also "Hidden Valley Ranch Dry Mix Products." Hidden Valley Ranch. Accessed October 31, 2013. http://www.cloroxprofessional.com/products/hidden-valley-ranch-dry/at-a-glance/.

Select Additional Sources
See pp. 626–629: Toussaint-Samat, Maguelonne. *A History of Food.* Oxford: Blackwell Publishing, 2009.
See chapter 2: *Agricultural Fact Book, 2001–2002.* U.S. Department of Agriculture, Office of Communications. Washington, DC: U.S. Government Printing Office, 2003.
"Fruit and Vegetable Consumption Among Adults—United States, 2005." *Centers for Disease Control and Prevention: Morbidity and Mortality Weekly Report.* Last updated March 15, 2007. http://www.cdc.gov/mmwr/preview/mmwrhtml/mm5610a2.htm.

Take-Out Reset
"To-go," which accounts for more than half the food
Horovitz, Bruce. "Takeout Takes Off." *USA Today.* Last updated June 13, 2007.
http://usatoday30.usatoday.com/educate/college/business/articles/20070617.htm.

dinner being the most popular
"Food for Thought." *U.S. Bureau of Labor Statistics.* Last updated November 2010.
http://www.bls.gov/spotlight/2010/food/.

little over $700,000 to open a restaurant
Huebsch, Russell. "The Startup Cost of Opening Restaurants." *Houston Chronicle*. Accessed October 31, 2013. http://smallbusiness. chron.com/startup-cost-opening-restaurants-1847.html.

about 60 percent of restaurants close
Hudgins, Catherine. "The Average Cost of Opening a Restaurant." *Houston Chronicle*. Accessed October 31, 2013. http://smallbusiness.chron.com/average-cost-opening-restaurant-14348.html.

In fact, according to a 2013 report
Lin, Biing-Hwan, and Guthrie, Joanne. "Nutritional Quality of Food Prepared at Home and Away From Home, 1977–2008." USDA Economic Research Service, Economic Information Bulletin no. 215 (2012).

launch of the TV dinner in 1953
See p. 162: McGinnis, J. Michael, Jennifer Appleton Gootman, and Vivica I. Kraak, eds. *Food Marketing to Children and Youth: Threat or Opportunity?* National Academies Press, 2006.

30 percent of our calories / 41 percent of our food dollar
Lin, Biing-Hwan, and Guthrie, Joanne. *Nutritional Quality of Food Prepared at Home and Away From Home, 1977–2008*. Economic Information Bulletin No. 105. U.S. Department of Agriculture, Economic Research Service, 2012.

Households that represent the highest 20 percent of incomes
"Food for Thought." U.S. Bureau of Labor Statistics. Last updated November 2010.
http://www.bls.gov/spotlight/2010/food/.

$660.5 billion industry
"Facts at a Glance." *National Restaurant Association*. Accessed October 31, 2103. http://www.restaurant.org/News-Research/Research/Facts-at-a-Glance.

not just fast-food but full-service restaurants as well
Stewart, Hayden, Noel Blisard, and Dean Jolliffe. *Let's Eat Out: Americans Weigh Taste, Convenience, and Nutrition*. No. 59411. U.S. Department of Agriculture, Economic Research Service, 2006.

In 1955, the same year / we spend nearly double that
Horovitz, Bruce. "Takeout Takes Off." USA Today. Last updated June 13, 2007.
http://usatoday30.usatoday.com/educate/college/business/articles/20070617.htm

typical American ate 81 meals in restaurants / 127 meals
Horovitz, Bruce. "Takeout Takes Off." *USA Today*. Last updated June 13, 2007.
http://usatoday30.usatoday.com/educate/college/business/articles/20070617.htm

take-out food comes with generous amounts of saltiness
Stewart, Hayden, Noel Blisard, and Dean Jolliffe. *Let's Eat Out: Americans Weigh Taste, Convenience, and Nutrition*. No. 59411. U.S. Department of Agriculture, Economic Research Service, 2006.
See also Appendix D: Henry, Jane E., and Christine L. Taylor, eds. *Strategies to Reduce Sodium Intake in the United States*. National Academies Press, 2010.
See also "Heart Attack Entrées and Side Orders of Stroke." Center for Science in the Public Interest. Last updated 2009. http://cspinet. org/new/pdf/cspirestaurantsaltreport.pdf.

full-service restaurants use more salt
Lin, Biing-Hwan, and Guthrie, Joanne. *Nutritional Quality of Food Prepared at Home and Away From Home, 1977–2008*. Economic Information Bulletin no. 105. U.S. Department of Agriculture, Economic Research Service, 2012.

Food scientists know the power of fat in flavoring
Gravitz, Lauren. "Food Science: Taste Bud Hackers." *Nature* 486, no. 7403 (2012): S14–S15.

take-out customers rank "taste" as the most important food
Stewart, Hayden, Noel Blisard, and Dean Jolliffe. *Let's Eat Out: Americans Weigh Taste, Convenience, and Nutrition*. No. 59411. U.S. Department of Agriculture, Economic Research Service, 2006.

Select Additional Sources
Kessler M.D., David. *The End of Overeating*. New York. Rodale, 2009.
See also Farley, Thomas A. "Salt Is a Problem; Salt Shakers Are." *New York Times: Room for Debate*. Last updated September 10, 2103. http://www.nytimes.com/roomfordebate/2013/09/10/should-salt-have-a-place-at-the-table/salt-is-a-problem-but-salt-shakers-arent.

Index

Recipe Index

Pooja's Select Product Picks

You'll find that a majority of the ingredients used in the Resets in this book can be found in farmers markets or CSA's (community-supported agriculture). Yet, there are some ingredients you'll use that can only be found in supermarkets or natural foods stores. Below are some of my favorite WAMP products. I've found these brands committed to making and/or sourcing the most sustainably made, delicious, whole and minimally processed products.

Sugar Reset

Grade A Maple Syrup from Whole Foods Market, wholefoodsmarket.com

Navitas Naturals Cacao Powder, navitasnaturals.com

TCHO Natural Cocoa Powder, tcho.com

Native Forest Organic Classic Coconut Milk (these are BPA-free cans), edwardandsons.com

Rapunzel Organic Whole Cane Sugar, amazon.com

Wholesome Sweeteners Organic Sucanat, wholesomesweeteners.com

Sweet Tree Organic Coconut Palm Sugar, bigtreefarms.com

Wedderspoon 100% Raw Premium Manuka Honey, wedderspoon.com

Salt Reset

Spectrum Toasted Sesame Oil, Unrefined, Organic, spectrumorganics.com

Eden Foods Organic Shoyu, Mirin, Rice Wine Vinegar, Soba Noodles, Sea Salt, Canned Kidney Beans, and Jarred Crushed Tomatoes, edenfoods.com

Organic Low-Sodium Beef Broth and Vegetable Broth, pacificfoods.com

Maine Sea Salt, maineseasalt.com

Celtic Sea Salt, celticseasalt.com

Wheat Reset

Kerrygold Grass-Fed Butter, kerrygoldusa.com

Whole Foods Market Organic Almond Milk, Unsweetened, wholefoodsmarket.com

Eden Organic Pinto Beans, edenfoods.com

Alter Eco Organic Quinoa, alterecofoods.com

Sweet Tree Organic Coconut Palm Sugar, bigtreefarms.com

Earthbound Farm Organic Baby Spinach, ebfarm.com

Nutiva Organic Virgin Coconut Oil, nutiva.com

Chocolate Reset

Theo Organic and Fair Trade Chocolate (70 percent cacao and above), theochocolate.com

Chocolate from The Chocolate Garage (70 percent cacao and above), thechocolategarage.com

Alter Eco "Dark Blackout" Bar, alterecofoods.com

Theo Chocolate Cacao Nibs, theochocolate.com

Navitas Naturals Cacao Nibs and Powder, navitasnaturals.com

TCHO Natural Cocoa Powder and PureNotes™ Dark "Chocolatey" 70%, tcho.com

Whole Foods Market Organic Almond Milk, Unsweetened, wholefoodsmarket.com

Saint Benoît Creamery Grass Fed Whole Milk, stbenoit.com

Straus Family Creamery Low Fat Grass Fed Milk, strausfamilycreamery.com

Yogurt Reset

Wallaby Organic Plain Low-Fat Yogurt and Greek Yogurt, wallabyyogurt.com

Stonyfield Organic Plain Yogurt, stonyfield.com

Saint Benoît Creamery Organic French-Style Yogurt (Grass Fed), stbenoit.com

Straus Family Creamery Organic Plain Whole and Nonfat Yogurt (Grass Fed),
    strausfamilycreamery.com

Chicken Reset

Marin Sun Farms Poultry, marinsunfarms.com

Find Pasture-Raised Chickens that can be shipped directly to you: localharvest.org

Beverages Reset

Numi Organic Loose Leaf Jasmine Green Tea, numitea.com

Rishi Tea Organic Jasmine Pearl Green Tea, rishi-tea.com

Rishi Tea Organic Golden Assam Black Tea, rishi-tea.com

Rishi Tea Organic Ancient Golden Yunnan, rishi-tea.com

Breakfast Reset

Alter Eco Organic Quinoa, alterecofoods.com

Whole Foods Market Organic Almond Milk, Unsweetened, wholefoodsmarket.com

Vital Farms Pasture-Raised Organic Eggs, vitalfarms.com

Bragg Liquid Aminos, bragg.com

Kerrygold Grass-Fed Butter, kerrygoldusa.com

Salad Reset

See my list for the *Salt Reset* above for Mirin and Shoyu brand picks

Eden Foods Organic Brown Rice Vinegar, edenfoods.com

Eden Foods Shiro Miso, edenfoods.com

Miso Master Organic Low-Salt Sweet White Miso, great-eastern-sun.com

South River Organic Sweet White Miso, southrivermiso.com

Earthbound Farm Organic Baby Arugula, ebfarm.com

Take-Out Reset

Nutiva Organic Virgin Coconut Oil, nutiva.com

Bragg Apple Cider Vinegar, Organic, Raw, Unfiltered,
   with the "Mother of Vinegar," bragg.com

Spectrum Toasted Sesame Oil, Unrefined, Organic, spectrumorganics.com

MiRancho Organic 100 Percent Corn Tortillas, miranchoretail.com

MaraNatha Organic Creamy Peanut Butter, maranathafoods.com

Arrowhead Mills Organic Peanut Butter, arrowheadmills.com

Acknowledgments

This book has been a labor of love that would not be possible without the support, trust, love, and dedication of so many.

To my husband, thank you for your infinite love, spirit, and commitment to this project. You are my sounding board and my bestie. To Valentina, the most precious gift of my life—thank you for bringing light, joy, and laughter into my every day. To Livia, your love and dedication to Vivi gave me the comfort I needed to make this book happen. To my father, for giving me the confidence, lust for life, and will to win from day one—I dream big because of you. To my bro, for being there no matter what and for your steadfast encouragement from the start. To Don and Linda, for your support and love—I am so thankful you both are in my life.

To Jane, You have made this book better with your unmatched attention to detail and wealth of talents. Thank you for being my right-hand.

To Kristyn, agent extraordinaire. You've been right beside me from inception— your dedication, trust, and loyalty are infectious. To the fabulous, bright, talented team of women who make up Seal Press—I couldn't have been luckier to have you as my publisher. To Domini, thank you for your passion and creativity—you have made this book beyond beautiful! I am so grateful for your efforts and hard work throughout. Laura, I couldn't think of being with a more intelligent, patient, and wise editor. To Eva, for your commitment to getting the word out and helping me share my work with the world—I can't wait to cook up more fun with you.

To Sunita at the Chocolate Garage, Dawn at Sustainable Table, and Joe and Debra at the incomparable Theo, for lending your ear and taking the time to review and support my work. Thanks to Slim & Sage for providing their lovely Pacific and Ruby dinner plates that make portion control and healthy eating feel effortless and luxurious through their fusion of science and fabulous design. Thanks, Tatyana!

And special thanks to Annemarie Colbin, Founder of NGI, and all of my teachers and mentors at the Natural Gourmet Institute—I have only you to blame for making me fall in love with health-supportive cooking and whole foods. You all have inspired me and taught me so much. I feel honored to have been guided by you.

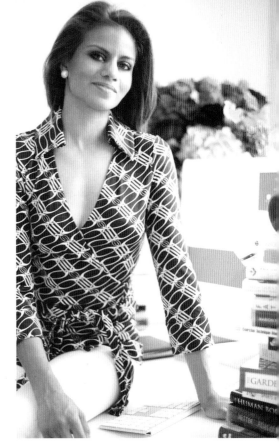

About
THE AUTHOR

Pooja Mottl is inspiring a conscious approach to healthy living in America. She is a Whole Foods chef, culinary instructor, healthy living speaker, and fitness and healthy-eating coach. A graduate of the Natural Gourmet Institute, she also holds a certificate in Plant Based Nutrition from Cornell University and a masters degree in international relations from the London School of Ecnomics. Pooja has appeared on *Good Morning America*, WGN-TV, *Martha Stewart Radio*, *The Huffington Post*, Style.com, the Green Festival, and many other media outlets. Pooja specializes in making healthy food delicious and simple to cook, and her food philosophy is based on the use of sustainable, organic, and unrefined ingredients to maximize flavor and nourishment. Her approach and tools have helped thousands of people experience a more vibrant life. Learn more about her at The3DayReset.com and PoojaMottl.com.